WELCOME TO YOUR NEW LIFE PLANNER!

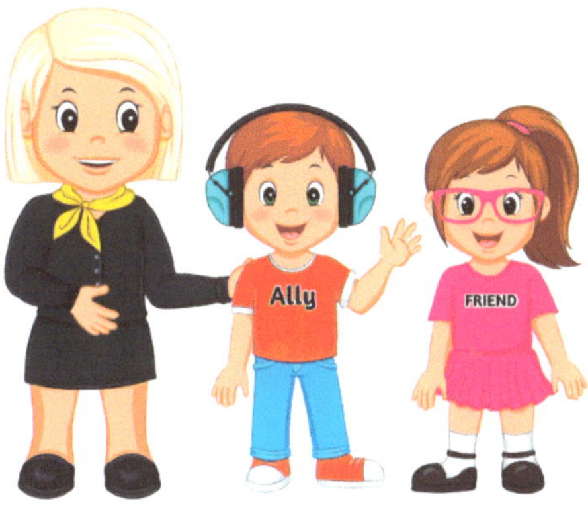

It's Ok Ally's "New Life Planner" is a personalized book to help parents, carers, and health professionals, set goals and milestones for special needs children, in order for them to live a balanced and well rounded life.

Most of what you see in your new life planner, will be square boxes, or ruled lines, across 30 different categories. The idea of the 30 categories is to emphasise that special needs children have the right to a balanced life - exactly the same as other family members too- however for this to occur, many times they will need extra supports to help them reach their goals, and in Australia, this is where NDIS funding comes in.

NDIS funding is a government support, that helps special needs kids gain extra supports in order to live life to their full potential, regardless of financial status. However to access this funding, you need to be able to state what the funding request for your child is, and why it is a necessity for your child's health and well being. Please note, NDIS funding is hard to receive, and can be a heartbreaking process to go through. It's my sincere hope that Ally's new life planner helps make the process a little [illegible] the outcome a little better, *before* your review.

itsokallyclipart   itsokallyclipart   itsokallyclipart

BECAUSE OF FUNDING RECEIVED LAST YEAR, I ACHIEVED THIS GOAL IN 12 MONTHS

Achievement: I got my hair cut at home by mum, and also at the hairdresser too!

Date this occurred: (Insert date)

How long it took me to reach my goal: (Insert months/days)

What resources helped me reach my goal? Mum brought me a social story book from itsokally.com for my ipad to read about getting my hair cut, and Zoe my OT did role playing practice sessions with me all year

This new skill has helped me be able to take pride in my appearance, tolerate people touching my hair, and not be afraid of different sounds at the hairdresser!

WELCOME TO YOUR NDiS GOALS AND MiLESTONE PLANNER!

Your "Goals and Milestone Planner" has been split into three sections to help you navigate forward with advocating for the special little people in your life.

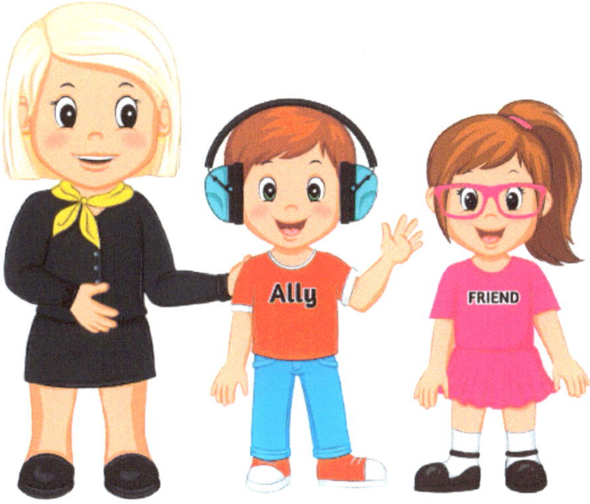

Part #1 is a daily routine planner, where you track and monitor your child's day and night for a week, to notice the places where they need help achieving regular goals and milestones that are integral to living a healthy balanced life.

Part #2 is your goals and supports tracker. This is where you identify the goals you believe your child needs to achieve to live a healthy balanced life, and in doing so, acknowledge the extra supports they need to help them achieve those specific goals.

And finally, part #3 offers basic health professional info, where you can put your health professional's details, and then fold and sticky tape copies of reports, to keep everything safe and all together.

CREATE YOUR OWN DAILY ROUTINE CHARTS

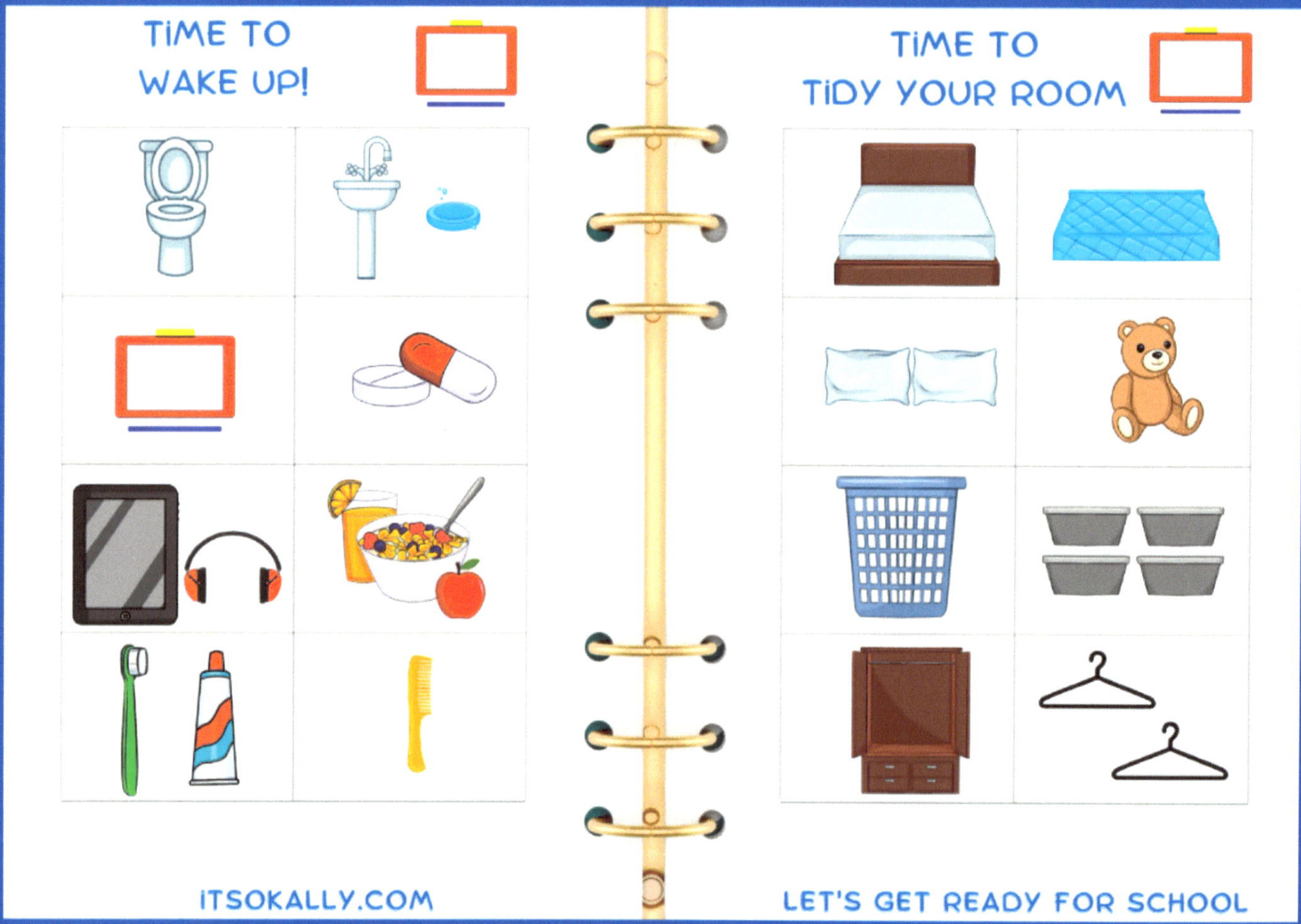

USE CLIPART, STICKERS OR WORDS!

ITSOKALLY.COM

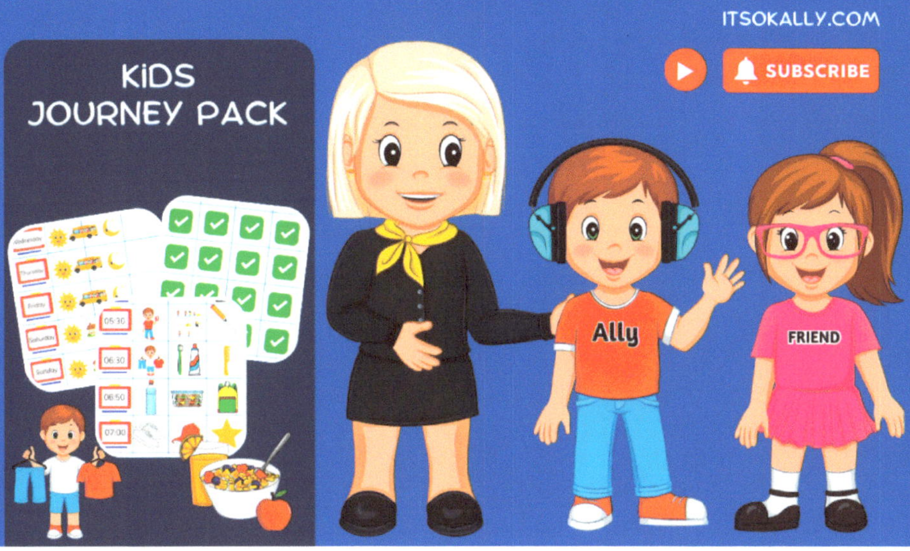

DOCUMENT YOUR ROUTiNE

If you are trying to get funding for your child's disabillity, then a recommended form of evidence/note taking is to keep a documented list of your child's routine.

Not only does this help you state your case in requesting extra help or supports, but it can also help parents/carers and support workers get a clearer view of where extra support is needed, along with the reasons why. To give you some examples of Ally's goals in 2023, I've listed some below:

- Getting Dressed independently (on his own)
- Brushing Teeth independently (on his own)
- Getting Ready For School independently (on his own)
- Having After Scool Calm Down Routine independently (on his own)
- Having Dinner, Bath, and Bed Routine independently (on his own)

Use the boxes on the following page to write down your child's weekly routine. When this section is finished, then move onto section #2. This is where you will document the goals you want your child to achieve and the supports you need to help facilitate this happening. If you need help, please feel free to reach out at: **itsokally.com**

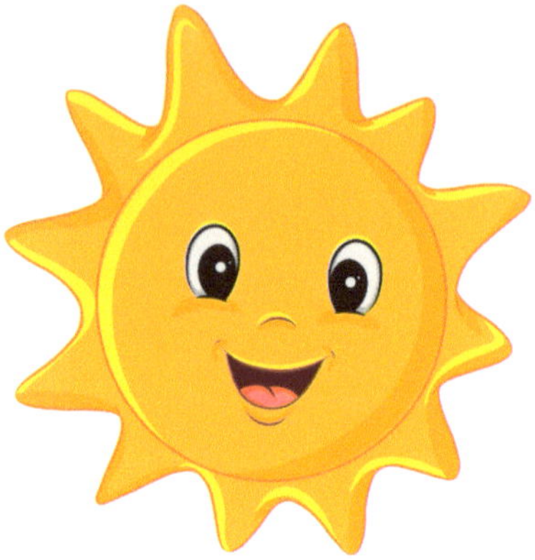

DAILY ROUTINE

MONDAY MORNING

DAILY ROUTINE

MONDAY MORNING

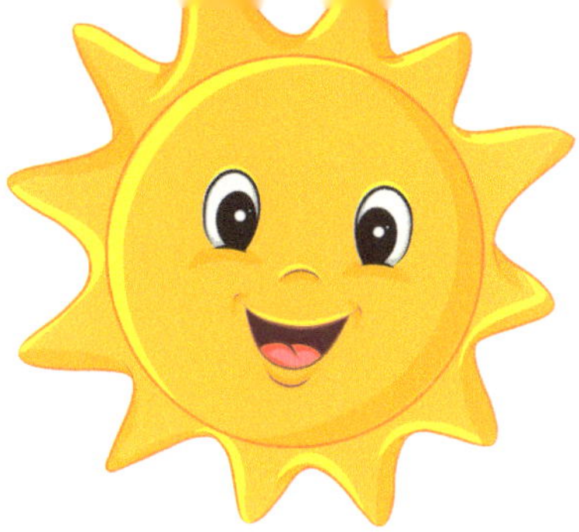

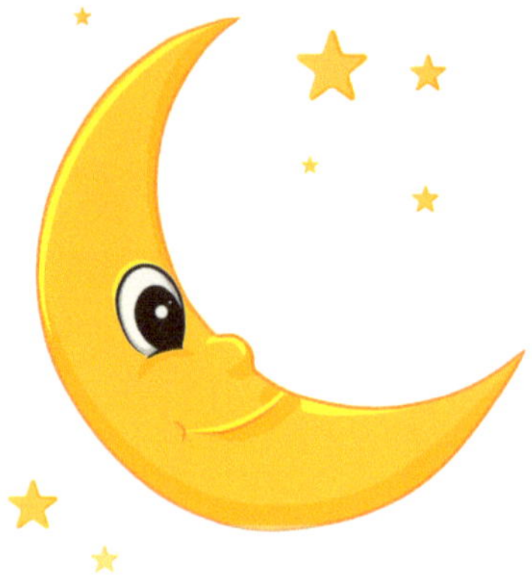

DAILY ROUTINE

MONDAY NIGHT

DAILY ROUTINE

MONDAY NIGHT

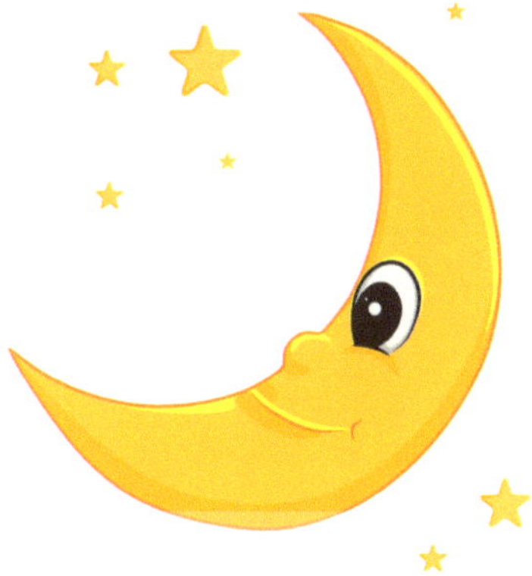

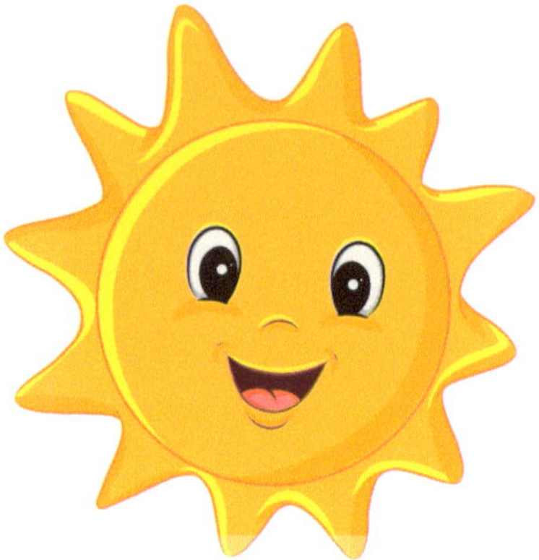

DAILY ROUTINE

TUESDAY MORNING

DAILY ROUTINE

TUESDAY MORNING

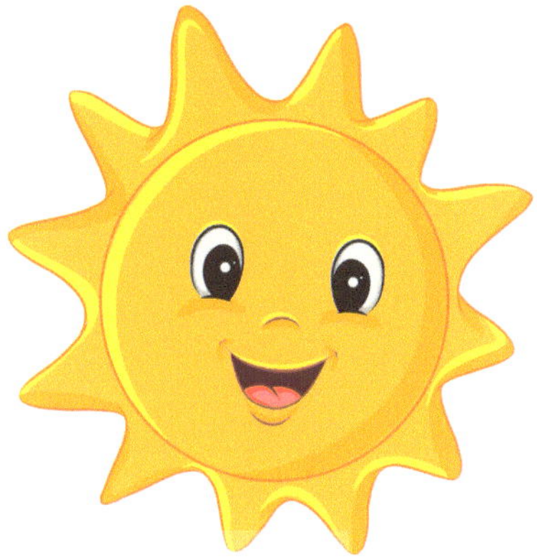

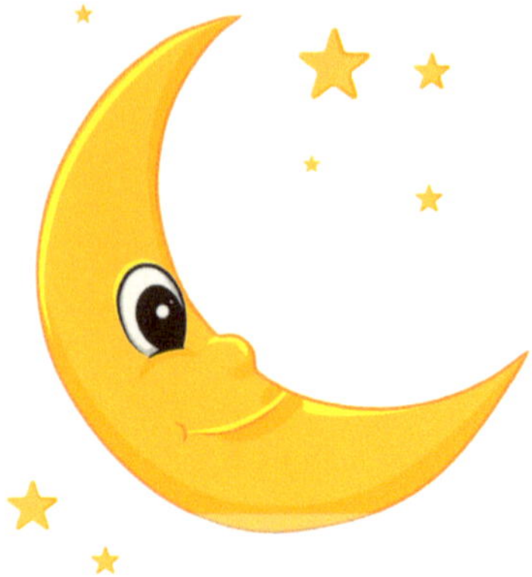

DAILY ROUTINE

TUESDAY NIGHT

DAILY ROUTINE

TUESDAY NIGHT

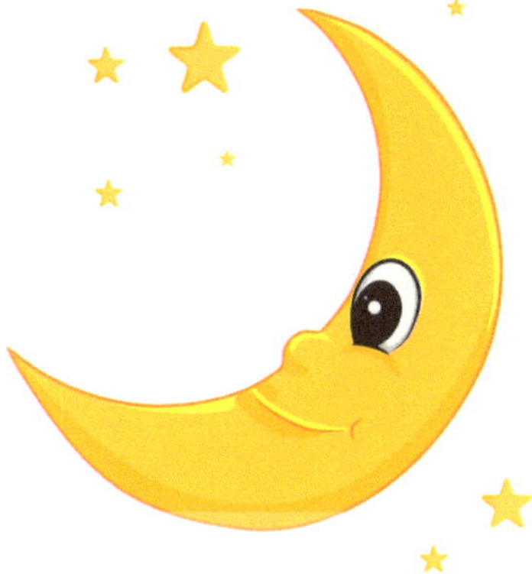

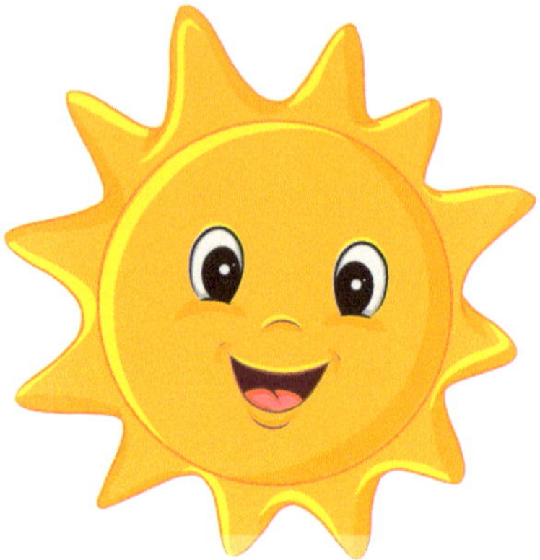

DAILY ROUTINE

WEDNESDAY MORNING

DAILY ROUTINE

WEDNESDAY MORNING

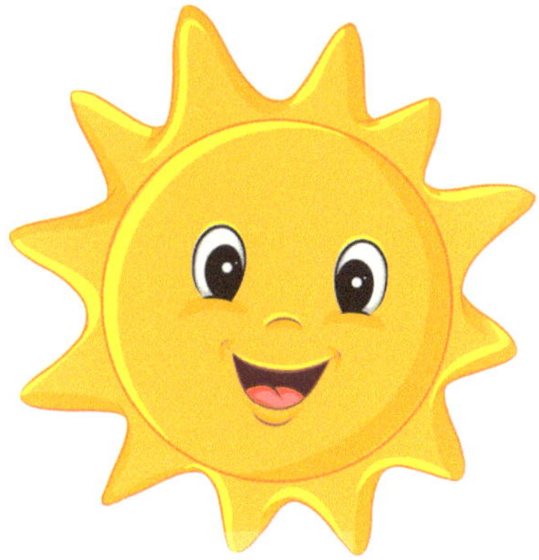

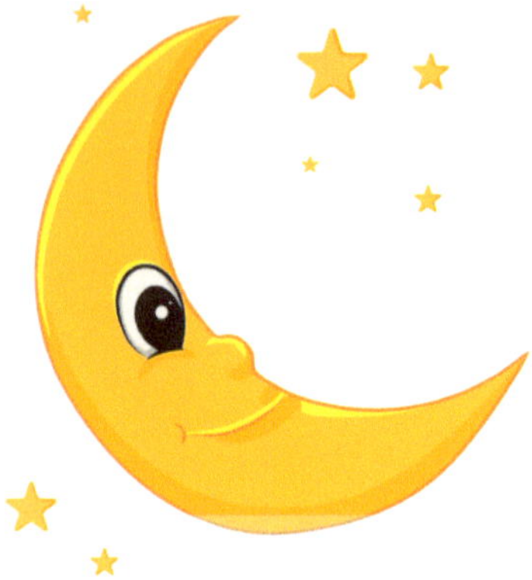

DAILY ROUTINE

WEDNESDAY NIGHT

DAILY ROUTINE

WEDNESDAY NIGHT

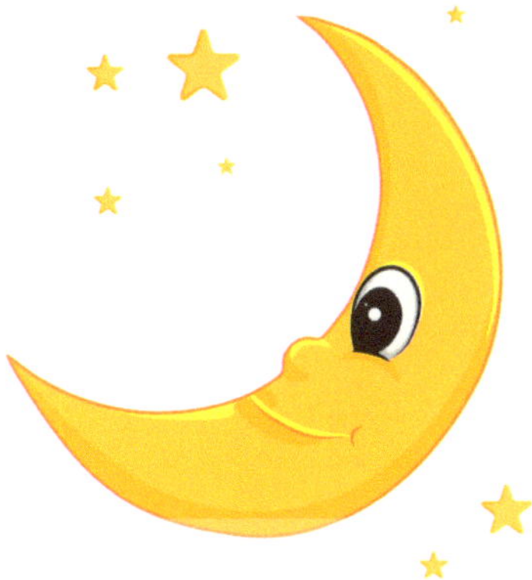

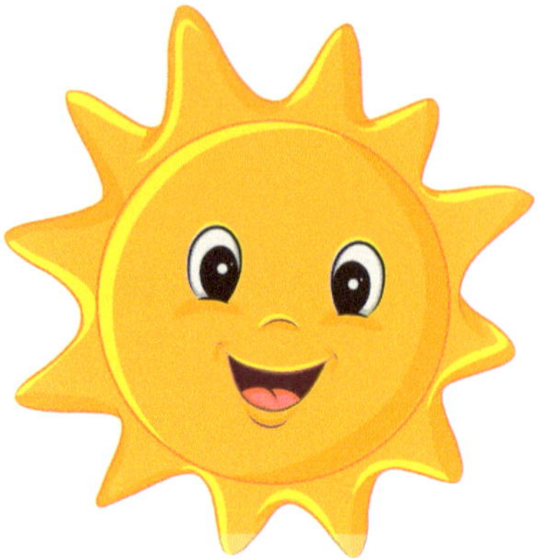

DAILY ROUTINE

THURSDAY MORNING

DAILY ROUTINE

THURSDAY MORNING

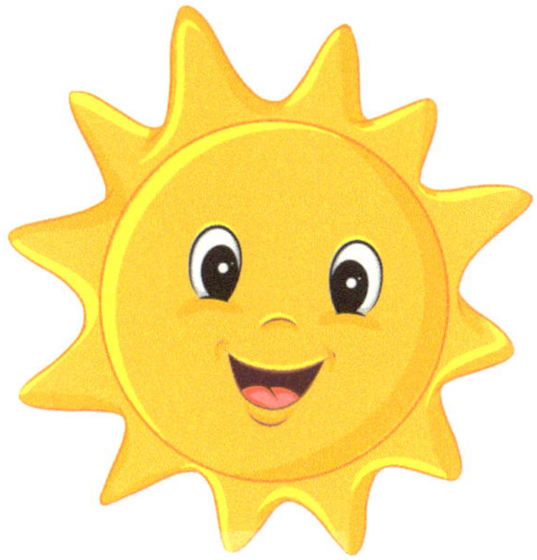

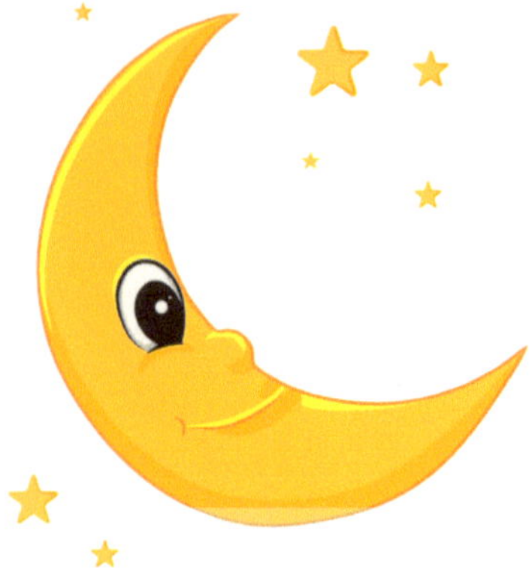

DAILY ROUTINE

THURSDAY NIGHT

DAILY ROUTINE

THURSDAY NIGHT

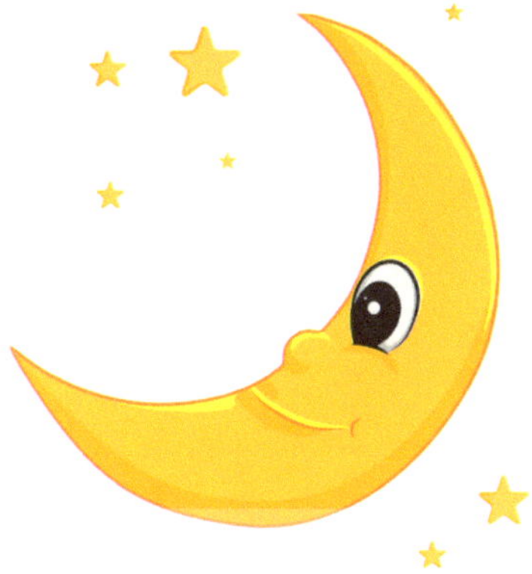

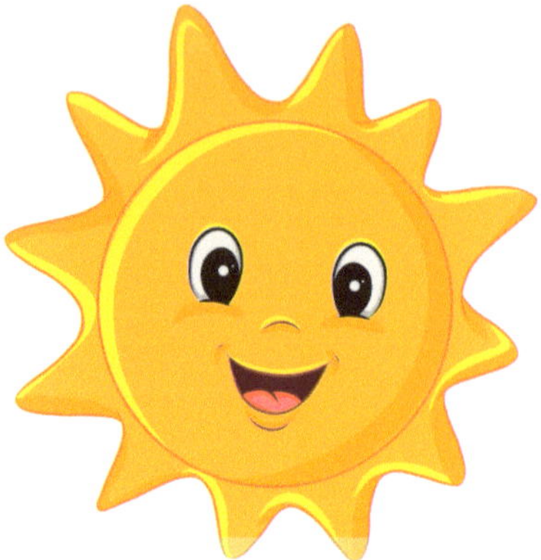

DAILY ROUTINE

FRIDAY MORNING

DAILY ROUTINE

FRIDAY MORNING

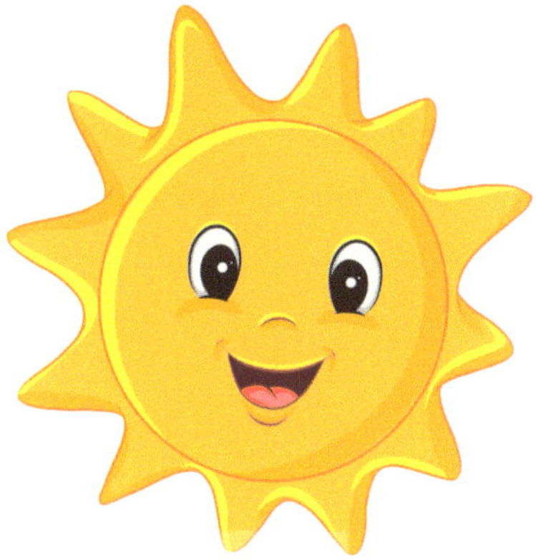

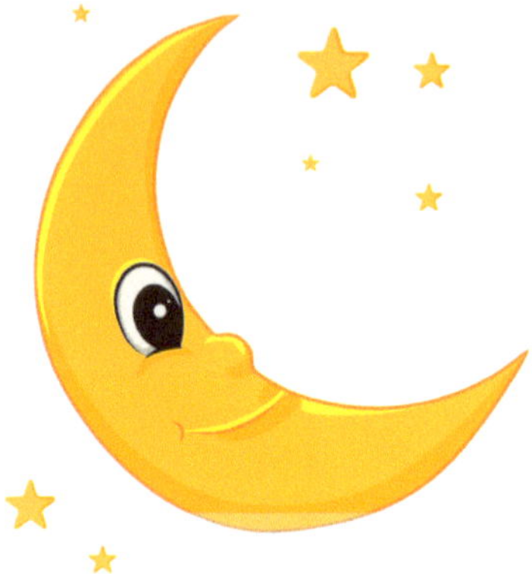

DAILY ROUTINE

FRIDAY NIGHT

DAILY ROUTINE

FRIDAY NIGHT

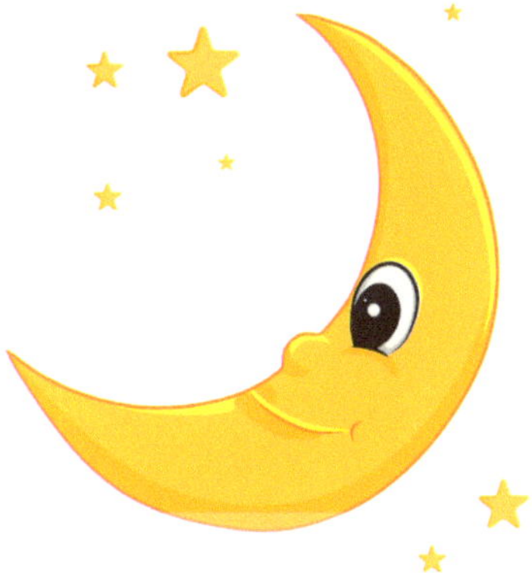

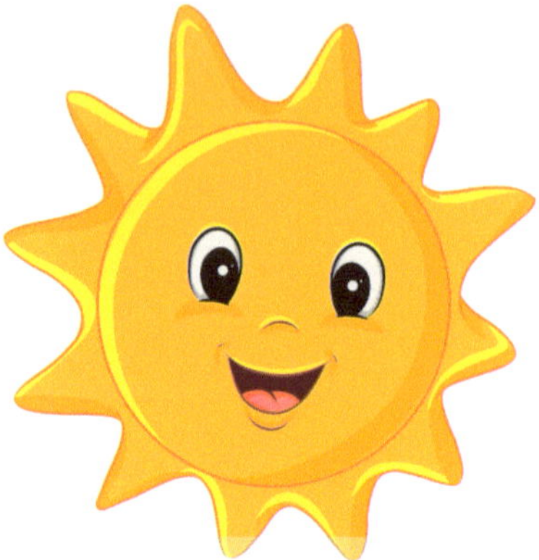

DAILY ROUTINE

SATURDAY MORNING

DAILY ROUTINE

SATURDAY MORNING

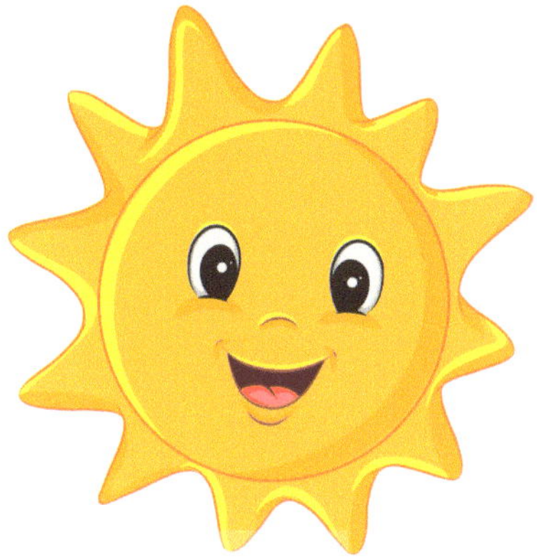

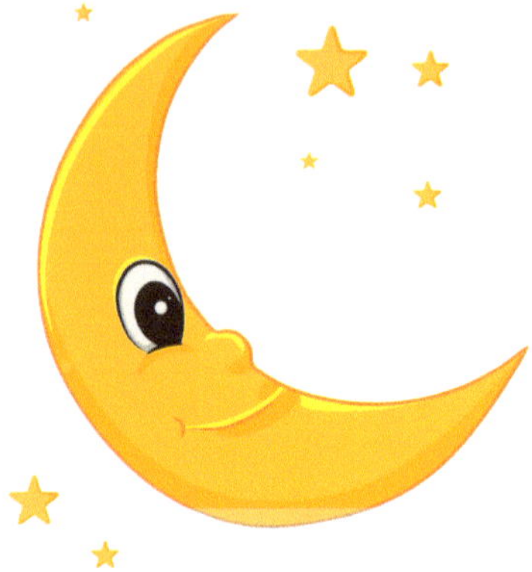

DAILY ROUTINE

SATURDAY NIGHT

DAILY ROUTINE

SATURDAY NIGHT

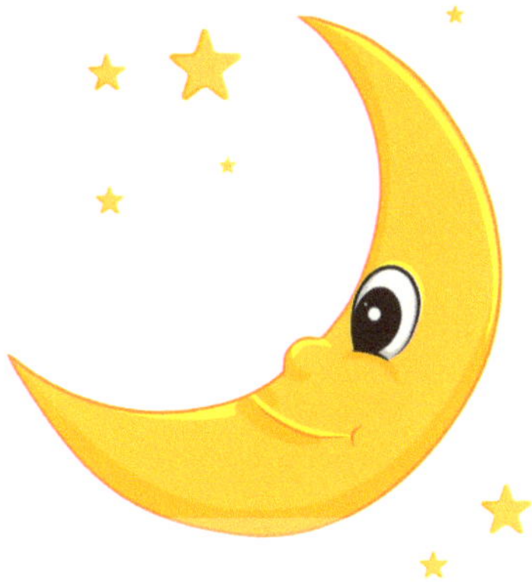

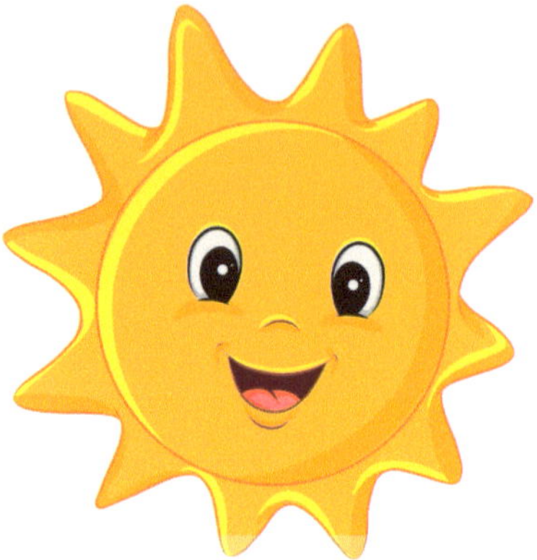

DAILY ROUTINE

SUNDAY MORNING

DAILY ROUTINE

SUNDAY MORNING

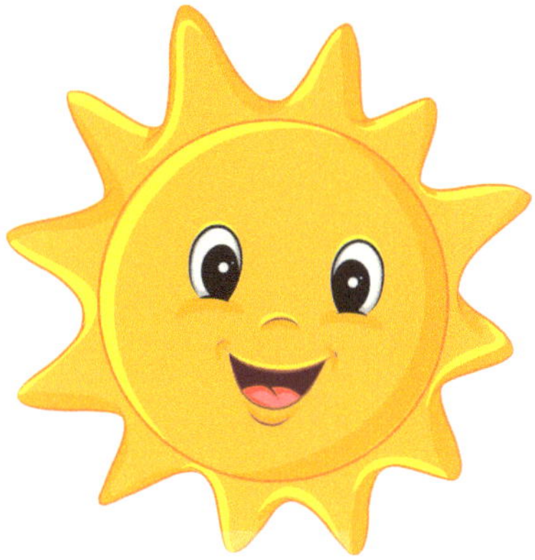

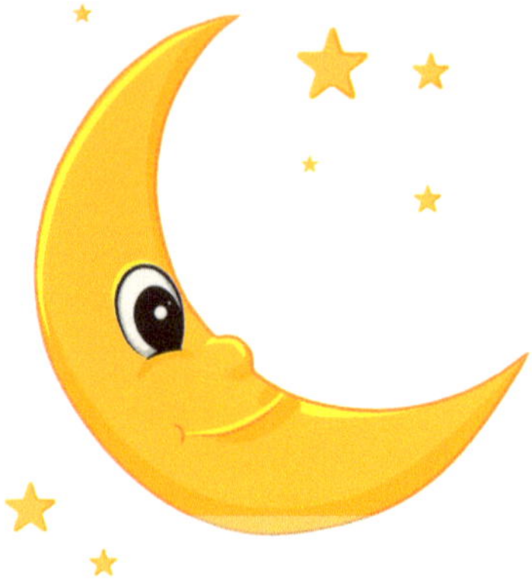

DAILY ROUTINE

SUNDAY NIGHT

DAILY ROUTINE

SUNDAY NIGHT

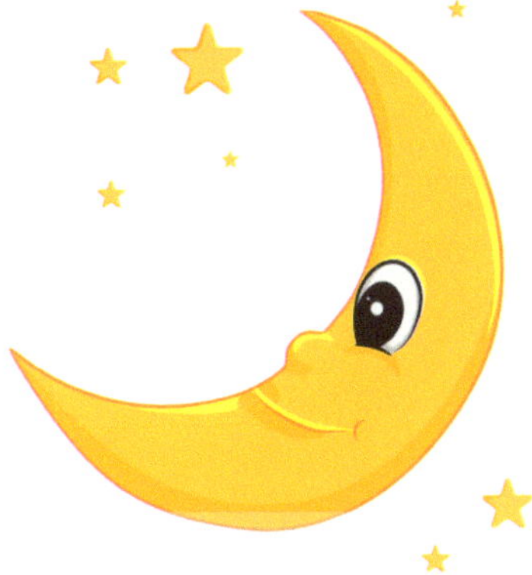

CREATE YOUR CHILD'S GOALS AND MILESTONES

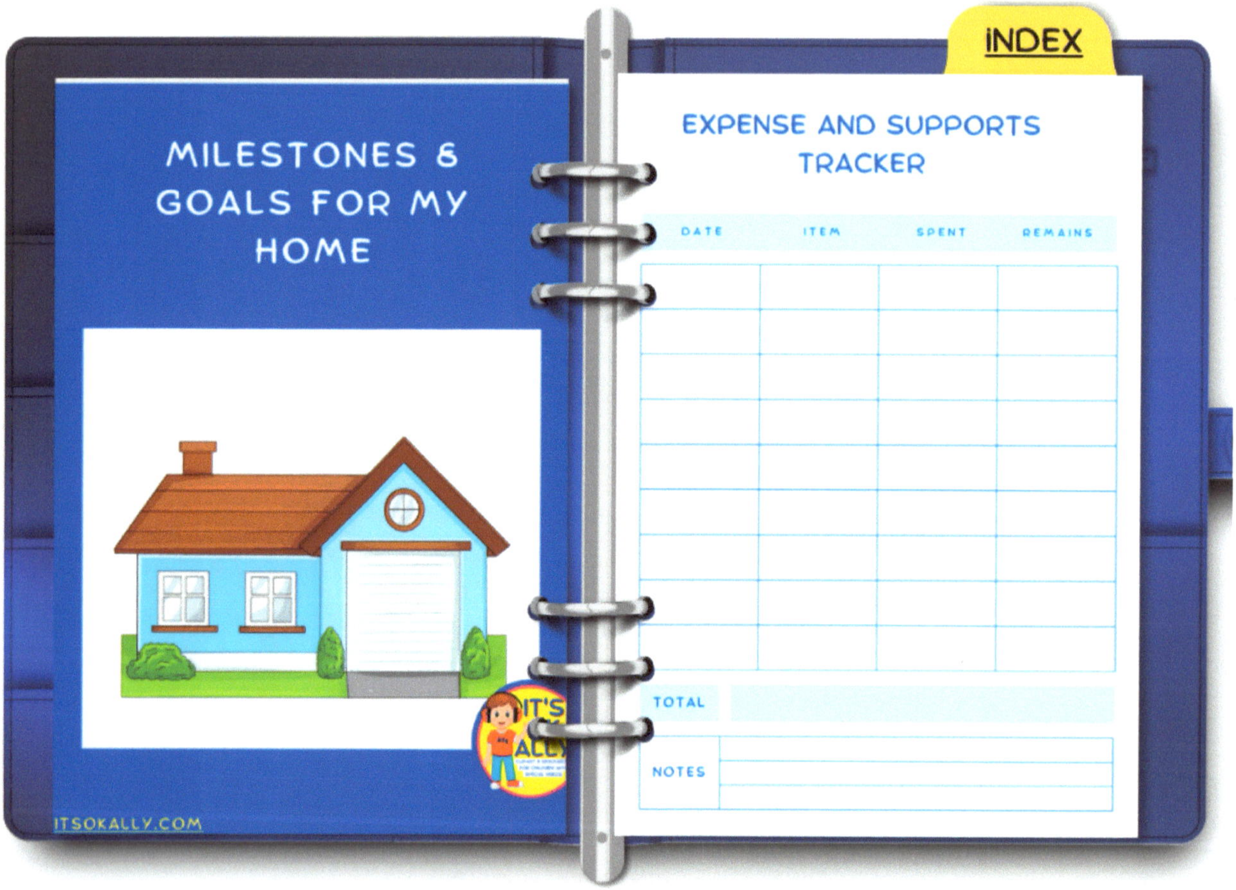

SET GOALS & TRACK MILESTONES & EXPENSES

ITSOKALLY.COM

DOCUMENT YOUR GOALS

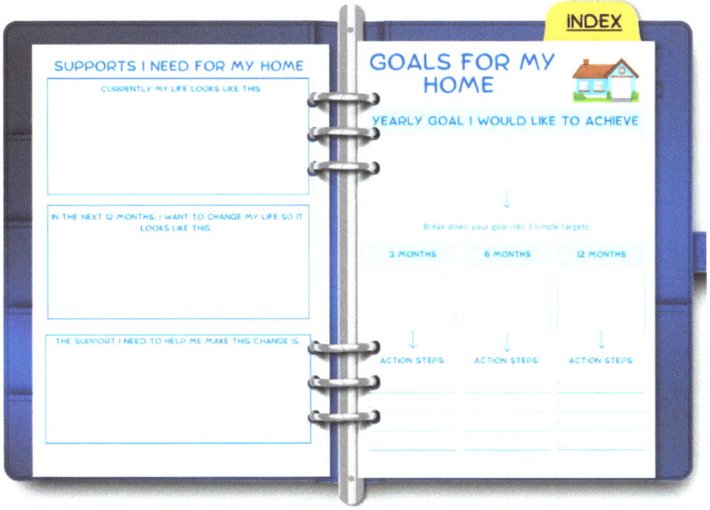

Once you have documented your child's weekly routine, the next thing to do is consider the goals you are advocating for your child, in order for them to live a healthy balanced life.

Although I have listed 30 categories for you, some of these categories may not apply at this exact moment in your child's development, and in this instance- just leave that specific category blank.

An example is Ally no longer needs supports or restrains for the car (he used to unbuckle his belt, and climb into the front of the car whilst I was driving or pull my hair to get my attention!) so our family won't fill in the car category this year.

Your family may not have pets or require a therapy dog, so you may leave this blank. Another family may not have a holiday house, simply leave this blank.

Once you become more familiar with my personal work (I do other journals aside from itsokally.com) you'll start to notice that we use these exact same 30 topics for kids, teens, and adults too, as I believe they form a strong foundation to live a balanced life.

MILESTONES & GOALS FOR MY HOME

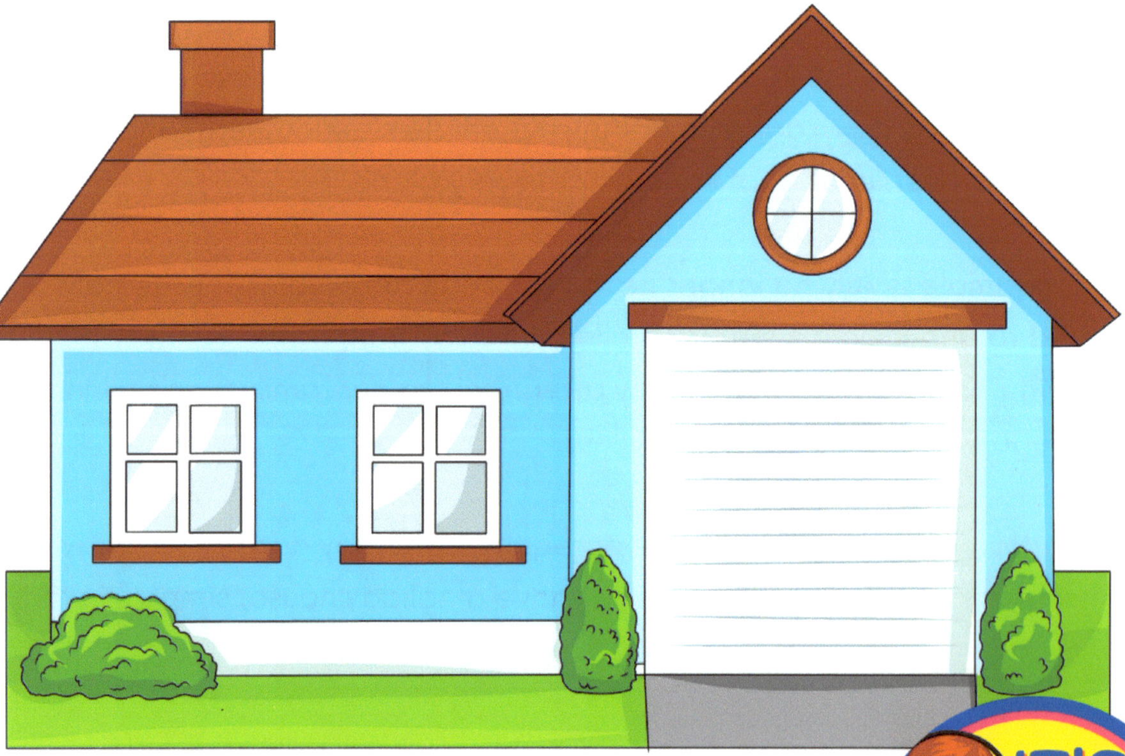

ITSOKALLY.COM

EXPENSE AND SUPPORTS TRACKER

DATE	ITEM	SPENT	REMAINS

TOTAL

NOTES	

SUPPORTS I NEED FOR MY HOME

CURRENTLY MY LIFE LOOKS LIKE THIS

IN THE NEXT 12 MONTHS, I WANT TO CHANGE MY LIFE SO IT LOOKS LIKE THIS:

THE SUPPORT I NEED TO HELP ME MAKE THIS CHANGE IS:

GOALS FOR MY HOME

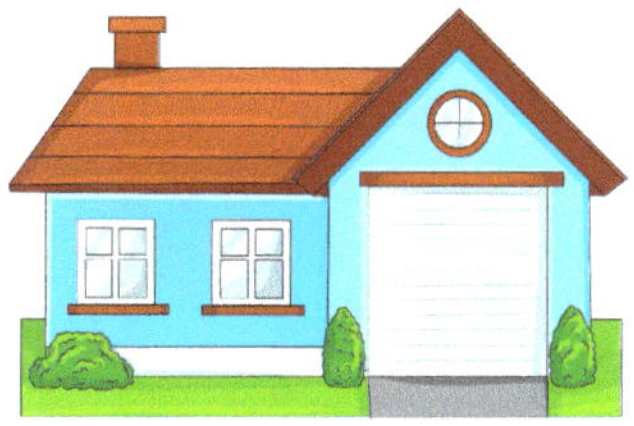

YEARLY GOAL I WOULD LIKE TO ACHIEVE

Break down your goal into 3 simple targets:

3 MONTHS	6 MONTHS	12 MONTHS
ACTION STEPS:	ACTION STEPS:	ACTION STEPS:
○	○	○
○	○	○
○	○	○
○	○	○

BECAUSE OF FUNDING RECEIVED LAST YEAR, I ACHIEVED THIS GOAL IN 12 MONTHS

Achievement:

Date this occurred:

How long it took me to reach my goal:

What resources helped me reach my goal?

This new skill has helped me:

THIS IS A PHOTO OF ME ON THE DAY I ACHIEVED MY GOAL

Use the Goodnotes "Add Image" button to add a photo of your achievement below

MILESTONES & GOALS FOR MY HEALTH

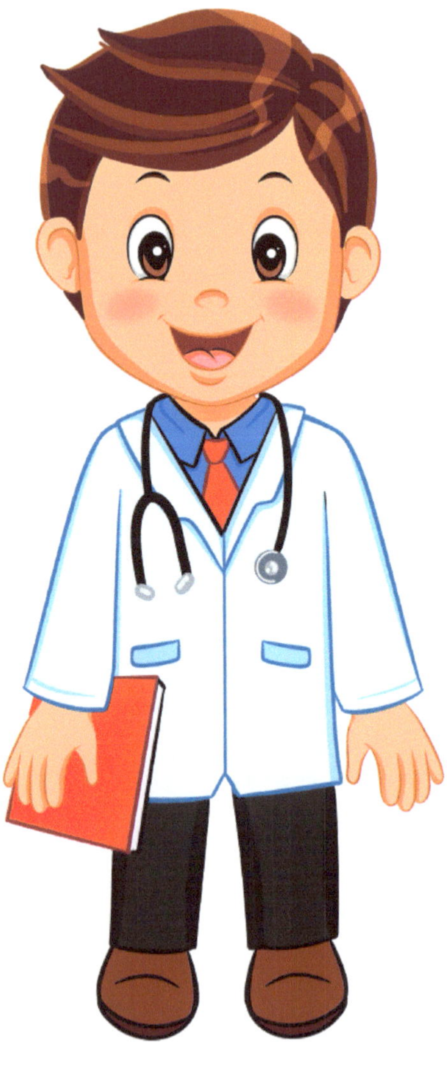

ITSOKALLY.COM

EXPENSE AND SUPPORTS TRACKER

DATE	ITEM	SPENT	REMAINS

TOTAL

NOTES	

SUPPORTS I NEED FOR MY HEALTH

CURRENTLY MY LIFE LOOKS LIKE THIS

IN THE NEXT 12 MONTHS, I WANT TO CHANGE MY LIFE SO IT LOOKS LIKE THIS:

THE SUPPORT I NEED TO HELP ME MAKE THIS CHANGE IS:

GOALS FOR MY HEALTH

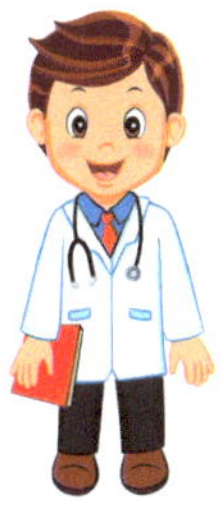

YEARLY GOAL I WOULD LIKE TO ACHIEVE

Break down your goal into 3 simple targets:

3 MONTHS	6 MONTHS	12 MONTHS
ACTION STEPS:	ACTION STEPS:	ACTION STEPS:
○	○	○
○	○	○
○	○	○
○	○	○

BECAUSE OF FUNDING RECEIVED LAST YEAR, I ACHIEVED THIS GOAL IN 12 MONTHS

Achievement:
Date this occurred:
How long it took me to reach my goal:
What resources helped me reach my goal?
This new skill has helped me:

THIS IS A PHOTO OF ME ON THE DAY I ACHIEVED MY GOAL

Use the Goodnotes "Add Image" button to add a photo of your achievement below

MILESTONES & GOALS FOR MY FITNESS

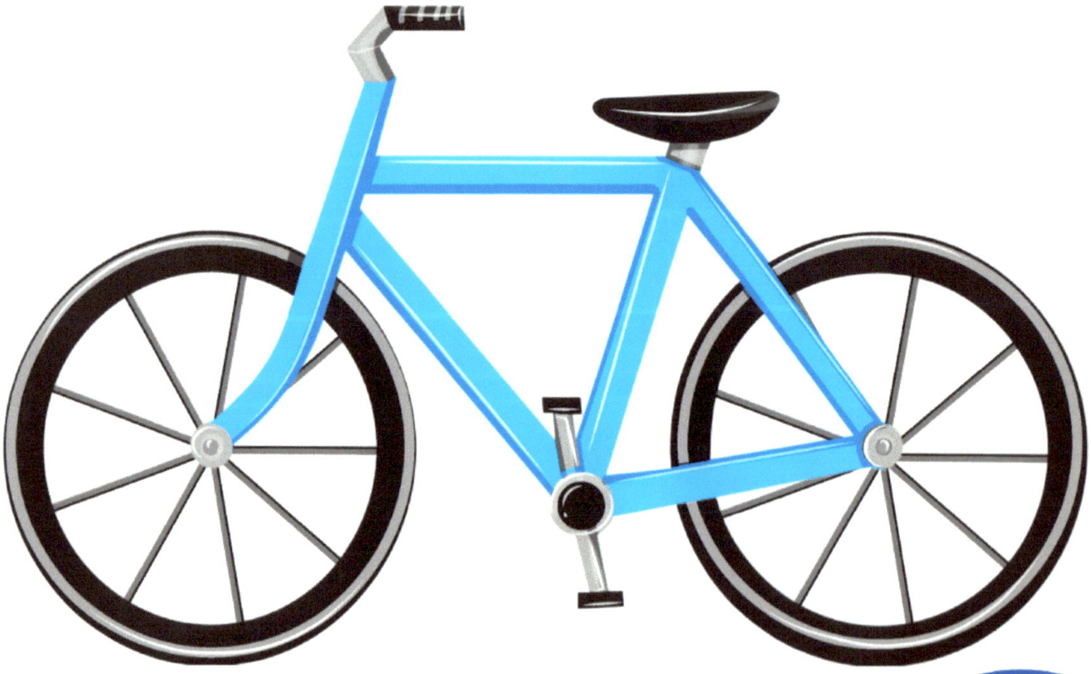

ITSOKALLY.COM

EXPENSE AND SUPPORTS TRACKER

DATE	ITEM	SPENT	REMAINS

TOTAL	

NOTES	

SUPPORTS I NEED FOR MY FITNESS

CURRENTLY MY LIFE LOOKS LIKE THIS

IN THE NEXT 12 MONTHS, I WANT TO CHANGE MY LIFE SO IT LOOKS LIKE THIS:

THE SUPPORT I NEED TO HELP ME MAKE THIS CHANGE IS:

GOALS FOR MY FITNESS

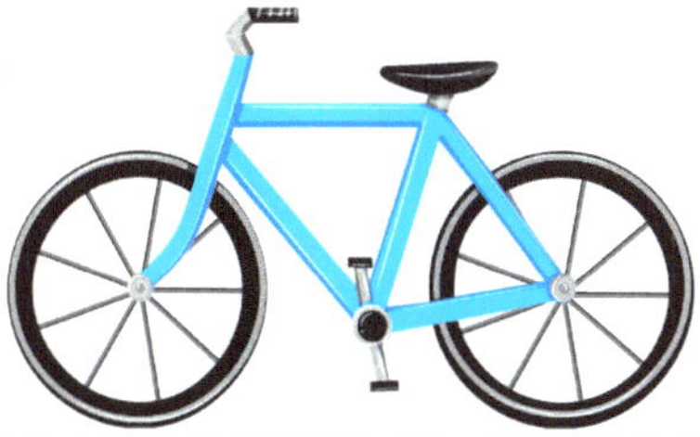

YEARLY GOAL I WOULD LIKE TO ACHIEVE

Break down your goal into 3 simple targets:

3 MONTHS	6 MONTHS	12 MONTHS
ACTION STEPS:	ACTION STEPS:	ACTION STEPS:
○	○	○
○	○	○
○	○	○
○	○	○

BECAUSE OF FUNDING RECEIVED LAST YEAR, I ACHIEVED THIS GOAL IN 12 MONTHS

Achievement:
Date this occurred:
How long it took me to reach my goal:
What resources helped me reach my goal?
This new skill has helped me:

THIS IS A PHOTO OF ME ON THE DAY I ACHIEVED MY GOAL

Use the Goodnotes "Add Image" button to add a photo of your achievement below

MILESTONES & GOALS FOR MY DIET

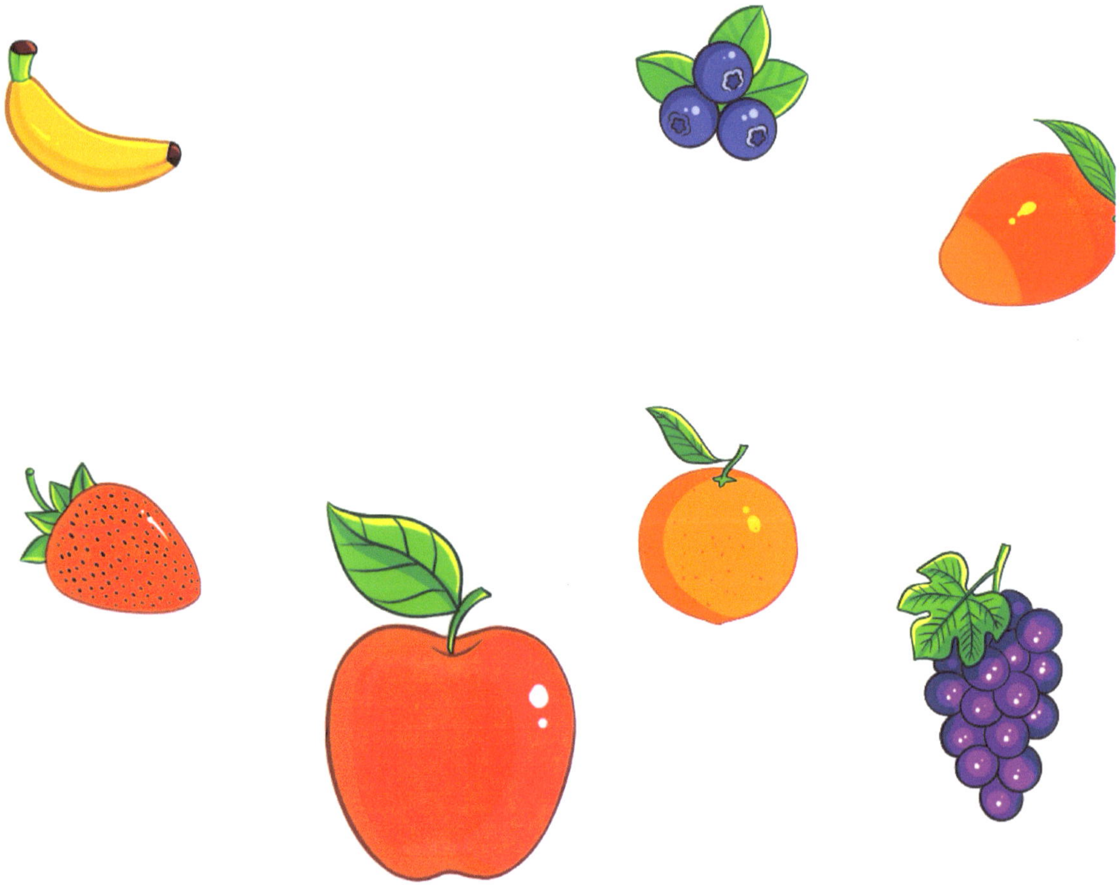

IT'S OK ALLY
CLIPART & RESOURCES FOR CHILDREN WITH SPECIAL NEEDS

ITSOKALLY.COM

EXPENSE AND SUPPORTS TRACKER

DATE	ITEM	SPENT	REMAINS

TOTAL

NOTES	

SUPPORTS I NEED FOR MY DIET

CURRENTLY MY LIFE LOOKS LIKE THIS

IN THE NEXT 12 MONTHS, I WANT TO CHANGE MY LIFE SO IT LOOKS LIKE THIS:

THE SUPPORT I NEED TO HELP ME MAKE THIS CHANGE IS:

GOALS FOR MY DIET

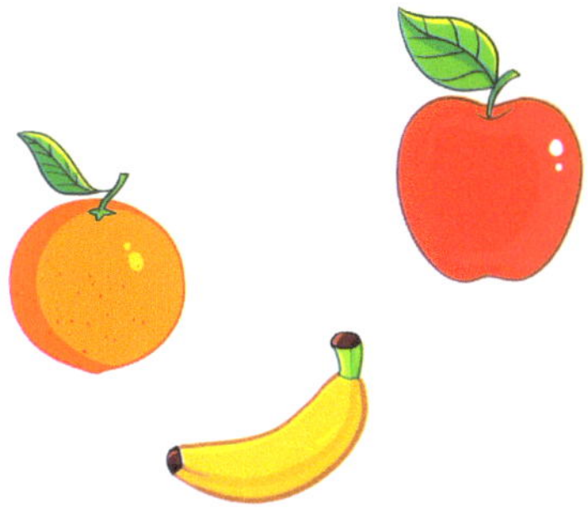

YEARLY GOAL I WOULD LIKE TO ACHIEVE

Break down your goal into 3 simple targets:

3 MONTHS	6 MONTHS	12 MONTHS
ACTION STEPS:	ACTION STEPS:	ACTION STEPS:

BECAUSE OF FUNDING RECEIVED LAST YEAR, I ACHIEVED THIS GOAL IN 12 MONTHS

Achievement:
Date this occurred:
How long it took me to reach my goal:
What resources helped me reach my goal?
This new skill has helped me:

THIS IS A PHOTO OF ME ON THE DAY I ACHIEVED MY GOAL

IT'S OK ALLY
CLIPART & RESOURCES FOR CHILDREN WITH SPECIAL NEEDS

Use the Goodnotes "Add Image" button to add a photo of your achievement below

MILESTONES & GOALS FOR MY MENTAL HEALTH

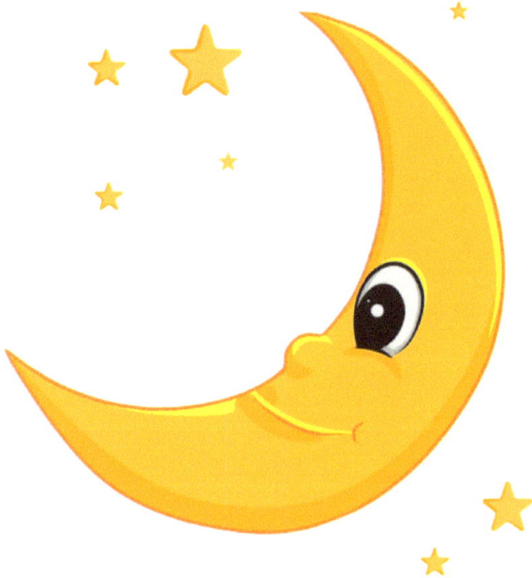

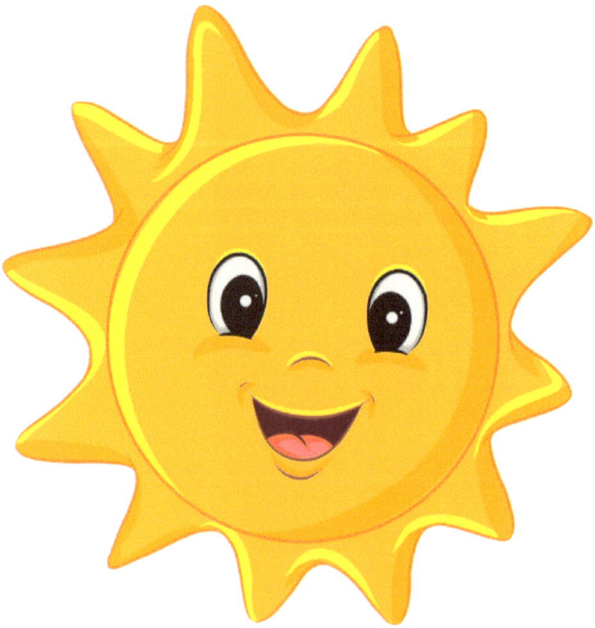

ITSOKALLY.COM

IT'S OK ALLY

CLIPART & RESOURCES FOR CHILDREN WITH SPECIAL NEEDS

EXPENSE AND SUPPORTS TRACKER

DATE	ITEM	SPENT	REMAINS

TOTAL

NOTES	

SUPPORTS I NEED FOR MY MENTAL HEALTH

CURRENTLY MY LIFE LOOKS LIKE THIS

IN THE NEXT 12 MONTHS, I WANT TO CHANGE MY LIFE SO IT LOOKS LIKE THIS:

THE SUPPORT I NEED TO HELP ME MAKE THIS CHANGE IS:

GOALS FOR MY MENTAL HEALTH

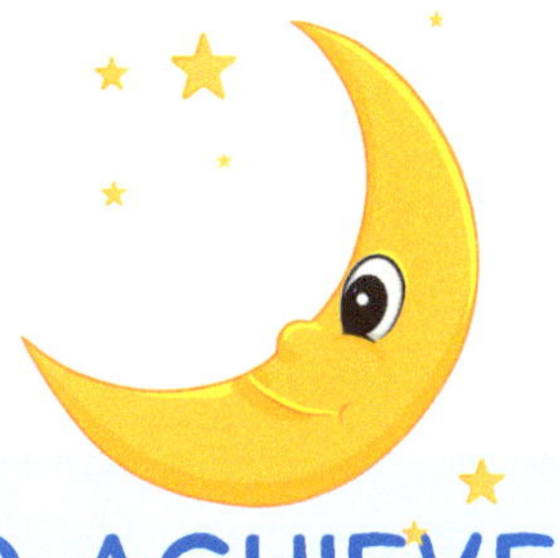

YEARLY GOAL I WOULD LIKE TO ACHIEVE

Break down your goal into 3 simple targets:

3 MONTHS	6 MONTHS	12 MONTHS

ACTION STEPS:	ACTION STEPS:	ACTION STEPS:
○	○	○
○	○	○
○	○	○
○	○	○

BECAUSE OF FUNDING RECEIVED LAST YEAR, I ACHIEVED THIS GOAL IN 12 MONTHS

Achievement:
Date this occurred:
How long it took me to reach my goal:
What resources helped me reach my goal?
This new skill has helped me:

THIS IS A PHOTO OF ME ON THE DAY I ACHIEVED MY GOAL

Use the Goodnotes "Add Image" button to add a photo of your achievement below

MILESTONES & GOALS FOR MY SELF CARE

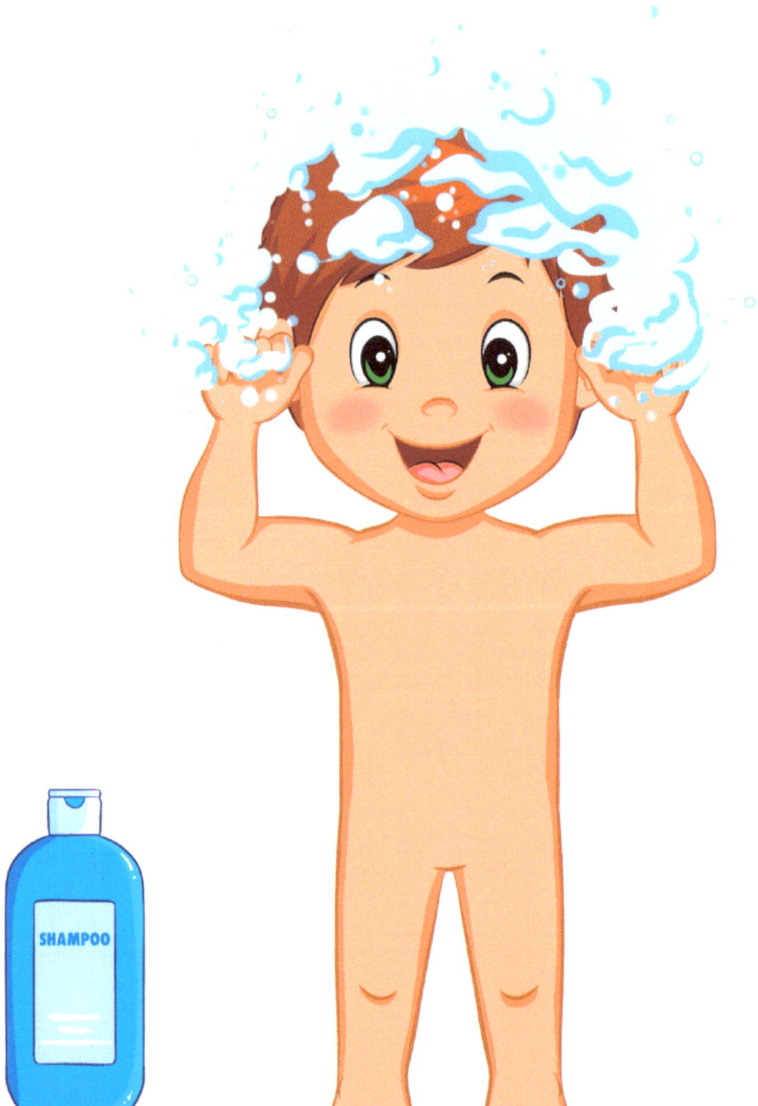

ITSOKALLY.COM

IT'S OK ALLY
CLIPART & RESOURCES FOR CHILDREN WITH SPECIAL NEEDS

EXPENSE AND SUPPORTS TRACKER

DATE	ITEM	SPENT	REMAINS

TOTAL

NOTES	

SUPPORTS I NEED FOR MY SELF CARE

CURRENTLY MY LIFE LOOKS LIKE THIS

IN THE NEXT 12 MONTHS, I WANT TO CHANGE MY LIFE SO IT LOOKS LIKE THIS:

THE SUPPORT I NEED TO HELP ME MAKE THIS CHANGE IS:

GOALS FOR MY SELF CARE

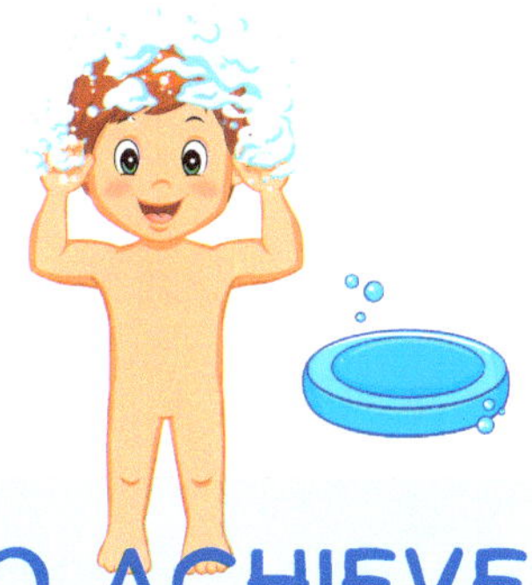

YEARLY GOAL I WOULD LIKE TO ACHIEVE

Break down your goal into 3 simple targets:

3 MONTHS	6 MONTHS	12 MONTHS

ACTION STEPS:

ACTION STEPS:

ACTION STEPS:

BECAUSE OF FUNDING RECEIVED LAST YEAR, I ACHIEVED THIS GOAL IN 12 MONTHS

Achievement:

Date this occurred:

How long it took me to reach my goal:

What resources helped me reach my goal?

This new skill has helped me:

THIS IS A PHOTO OF ME ON THE DAY I ACHIEVED MY GOAL

Use the Goodnotes "Add Image" button to add a photo of your achievement below

MILESTONES & GOALS FOR MY MINDFULNESS

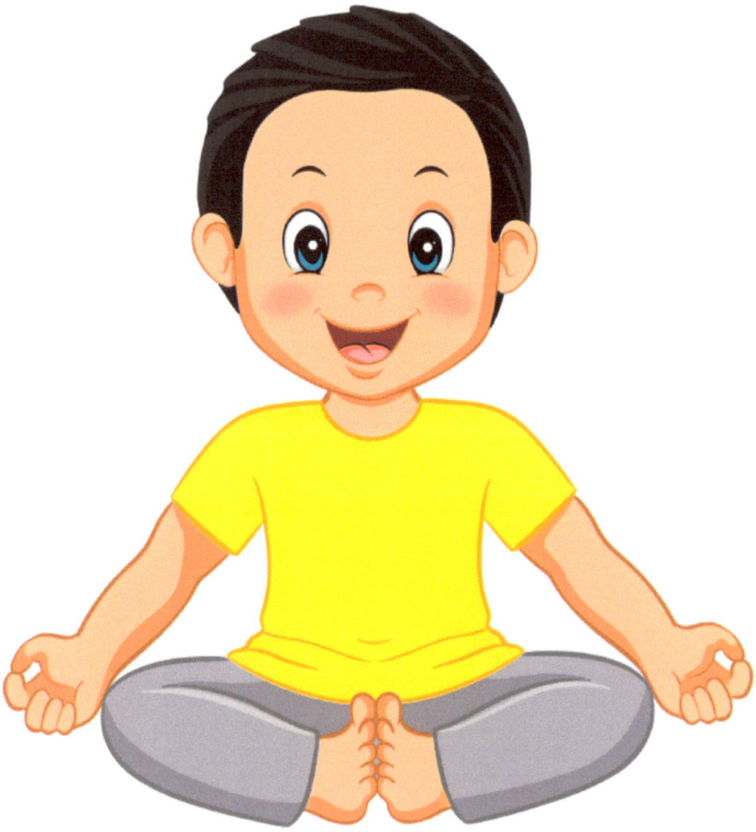

ITSOKALLY.COM

EXPENSE AND SUPPORTS TRACKER

DATE	ITEM	SPENT	REMAINS

TOTAL

NOTES	

SUPPORTS I NEED FOR MY MINDFULNESS

CURRENTLY MY LIFE LOOKS LIKE THIS

IN THE NEXT 12 MONTHS, I WANT TO CHANGE MY LIFE SO IT LOOKS LIKE THIS:

THE SUPPORT I NEED TO HELP ME MAKE THIS CHANGE IS:

GOALS FOR MY MINDFULNESS

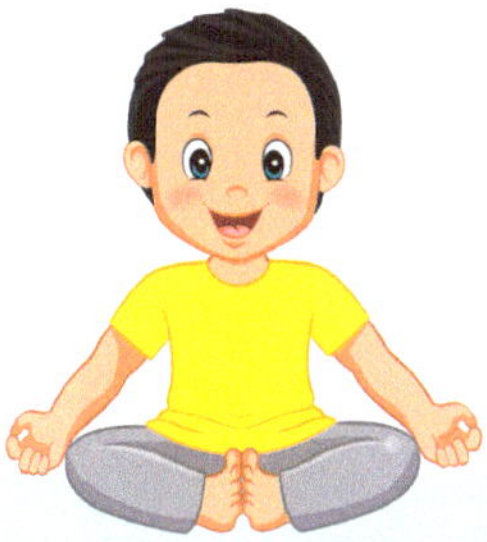

YEARLY GOAL I WOULD LIKE TO ACHIEVE

Break down your goal into 3 simple targets:

3 MONTHS	6 MONTHS	12 MONTHS
ACTION STEPS:	ACTION STEPS:	ACTION STEPS:

BECAUSE OF FUNDING RECEIVED LAST YEAR, I ACHIEVED THIS GOAL IN 12 MONTHS

Achievement:
Date this occurred:
How long it took me to reach my goal:
What resources helped me reach my goal?
This new skill has helped me:

THIS IS A PHOTO OF ME ON THE DAY I ACHIEVED MY GOAL

Use the Goodnotes "Add Image" button to add a photo of your achievement below

MILESTONES & GOALS FOR MY VIRTUES

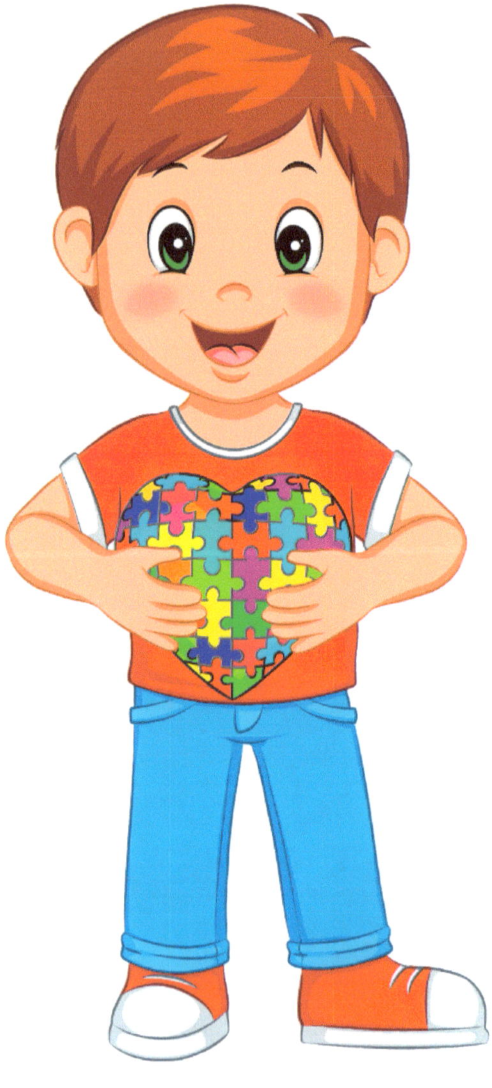

EXPENSE AND SUPPORTS TRACKER

DATE	ITEM	SPENT	REMAINS

TOTAL

NOTES	

SUPPORTS I NEED FOR MY VIRTUES

CURRENTLY MY LIFE LOOKS LIKE THIS

IN THE NEXT 12 MONTHS, I WANT TO CHANGE MY LIFE SO IT LOOKS LIKE THIS:

THE SUPPORT I NEED TO HELP ME MAKE THIS CHANGE IS:

GOALS FOR MY VIRTUES

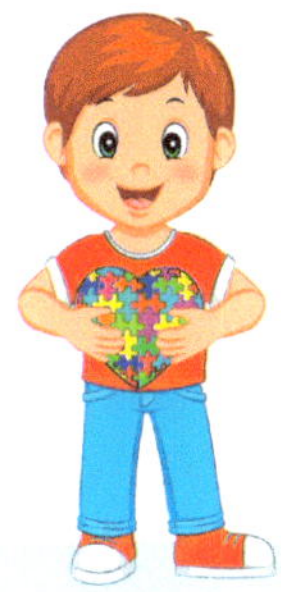

YEARLY GOAL I WOULD LIKE TO ACHIEVE

Break down your goal into 3 simple targets:

3 MONTHS	6 MONTHS	12 MONTHS
ACTION STEPS:	ACTION STEPS:	ACTION STEPS:

BECAUSE OF FUNDING RECEIVED LAST YEAR, I ACHIEVED THIS GOAL IN 12 MONTHS

Achievement:
Date this occurred:
How long it took me to reach my goal:
What resources helped me reach my goal?
This new skill has helped me:

THIS IS A PHOTO OF ME ON THE DAY I ACHIEVED MY GOAL

Use the Goodnotes "Add Image" button to add a photo of your achievement below

MILESTONES & GOALS FOR MY ITEMS OF VALUE

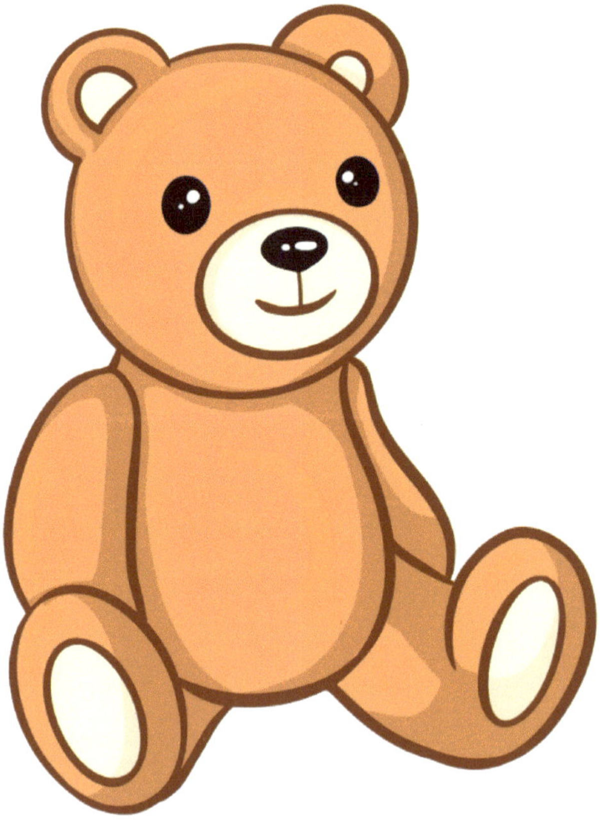

ITSOKALLY.COM

EXPENSE AND SUPPORTS TRACKER

DATE	ITEM	SPENT	REMAINS

TOTAL

NOTES	

SUPPORTS I NEED FOR MY ITEMS OF VALUE

CURRENTLY MY LIFE LOOKS LIKE THIS

IN THE NEXT 12 MONTHS, I WANT TO CHANGE MY LIFE SO IT LOOKS LIKE THIS:

THE SUPPORT I NEED TO HELP ME MAKE THIS CHANGE IS:

GOALS FOR MY ITEMS OF VALUE

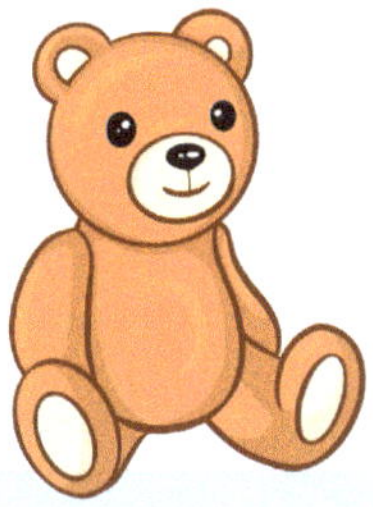

YEARLY GOAL I WOULD LIKE TO ACHIEVE

Break down your goal into 3 simple targets:

3 MONTHS	6 MONTHS	12 MONTHS

ACTION STEPS:

ACTION STEPS:

ACTION STEPS:

BECAUSE OF FUNDING RECEIVED LAST YEAR, I ACHIEVED THIS GOAL IN 12 MONTHS

Achievement:
Date this occurred:
How long it took me to reach my goal:
What resources helped me reach my goal?
This new skill has helped me:

THIS IS A PHOTO OF ME ON THE DAY I ACHIEVED MY GOAL

Use the Goodnotes "Add Image" button to add a photo of your achievement below

MILESTONES & GOALS FOR MY FAMILY

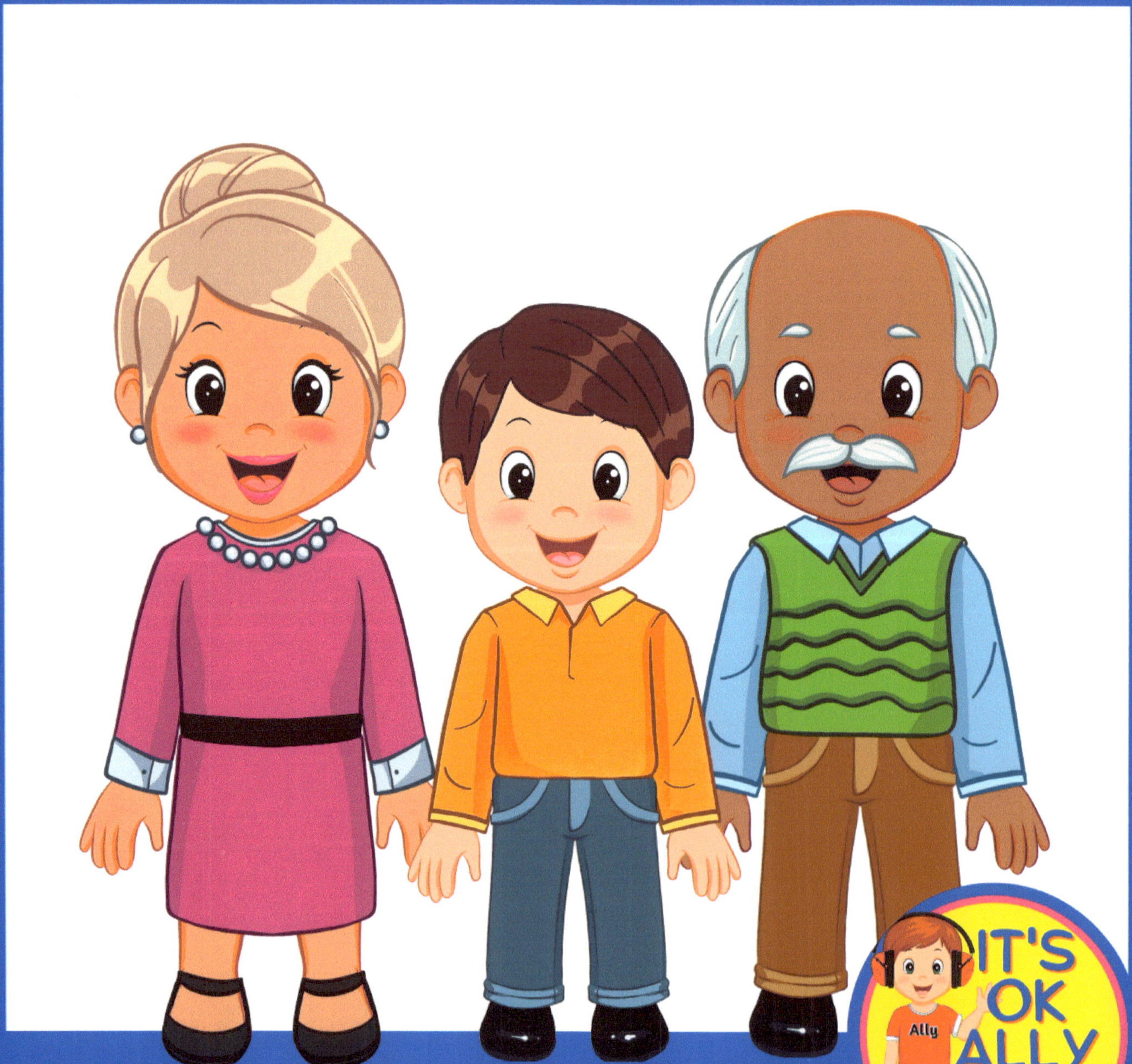

ITSOKALLY.COM

EXPENSE AND SUPPORTS TRACKER

DATE	ITEM	SPENT	REMAINS

TOTAL

NOTES	

GOALS FOR MY FAMiLY

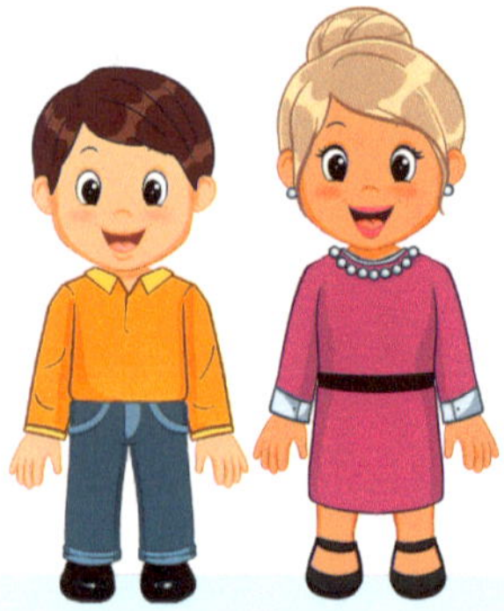

YEARLY GOAL I WOULD LIKE TO ACHIEVE

Break down your goal into 3 simple targets:

3 MONTHS	6 MONTHS	12 MONTHS
ACTiON STEPS:	ACTiON STEPS:	ACTiON STEPS:

SUPPORTS I NEED FOR MY FAMILY

CURRENTLY MY LIFE LOOKS LIKE THIS

IN THE NEXT 12 MONTHS, I WANT TO CHANGE MY LIFE SO IT LOOKS LIKE THIS:

THE SUPPORT I NEED TO HELP ME MAKE THIS CHANGE IS:

BECAUSE OF FUNDING RECEIVED LAST YEAR, I ACHIEVED THIS GOAL IN 12 MONTHS

IT'S OK ALLY
CLIPART & RESOURCES FOR CHILDREN WITH SPECIAL NEEDS

Achievement:
Date this occurred:
How long it took me to reach my goal:
What resources helped me reach my goal?
This new skill has helped me:

THIS IS A PHOTO OF ME ON THE DAY I ACHIEVED MY GOAL

Use the Goodnotes "Add Image" button to add a photo of your achievement below

MILESTONES & GOALS FOR MY FRIENDSHIPS

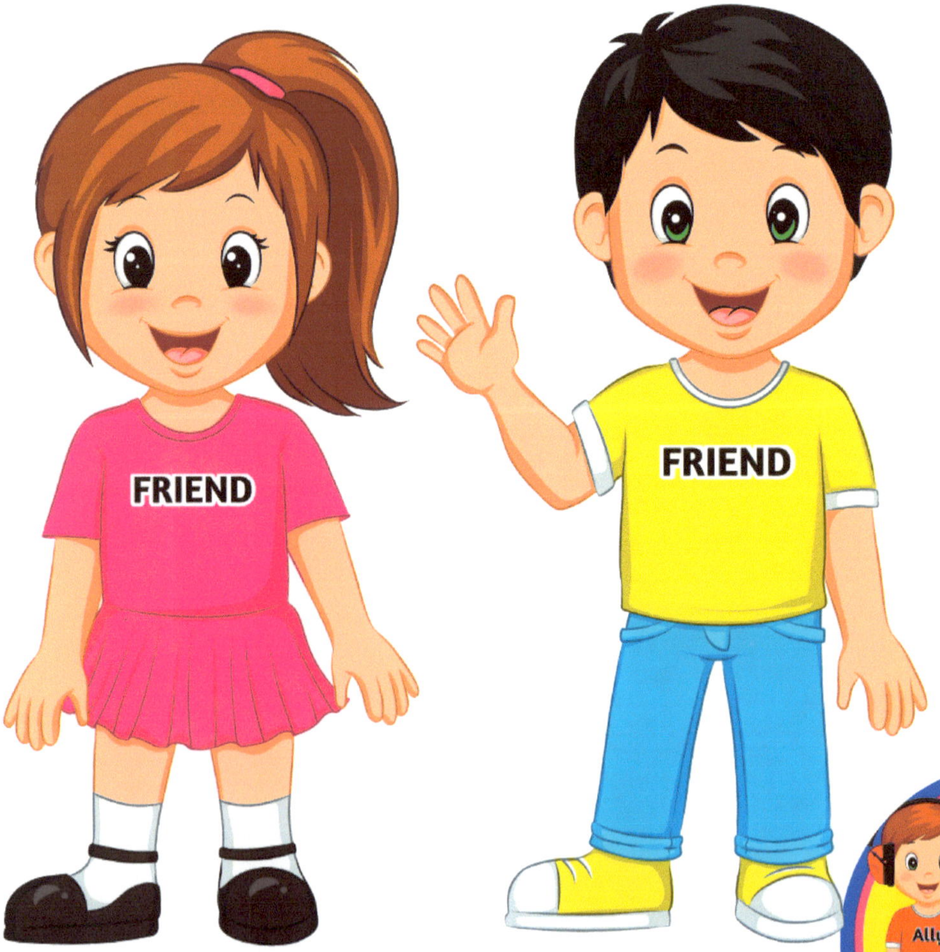

ITSOKALLY.COM

CLIPART & RESOURCES FOR CHILDREN WITH SPECIAL NEEDS

EXPENSE AND SUPPORTS TRACKER

DATE	ITEM	SPENT	REMAINS

TOTAL

NOTES	

SUPPORTS I NEED FOR MY FRIENDSHIPS

CURRENTLY MY LIFE LOOKS LIKE THIS

IN THE NEXT 12 MONTHS, I WANT TO CHANGE MY LIFE SO IT LOOKS LIKE THIS:

THE SUPPORT I NEED TO HELP ME MAKE THIS CHANGE IS:

GOALS FOR MY FRIENDSHIPS

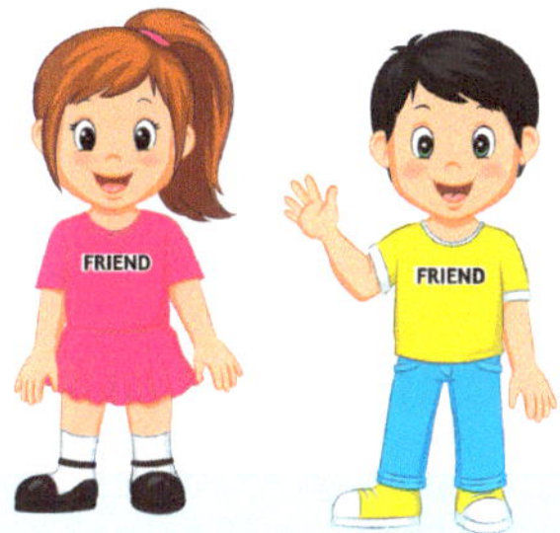

YEARLY GOAL I WOULD LIKE TO ACHIEVE

Break down your goal into 3 simple targets:

3 MONTHS	6 MONTHS	12 MONTHS

ACTION STEPS:	ACTION STEPS:	ACTION STEPS:
○	○	○
○	○	○
○	○	○
○	○	○

BECAUSE OF FUNDING RECEIVED LAST YEAR, I ACHIEVED THIS GOAL IN 12 MONTHS

IT'S OK ALLY
CLIPART & RESOURCES FOR CHILDREN WITH SPECIAL NEEDS

Achievement:
Date this occurred:
How long it took me to reach my goal:
What resources helped me reach my goal?
This new skill has helped me:

THIS IS A PHOTO OF ME ON THE DAY I ACHIEVED MY GOAL

Use the Goodnotes "Add Image" button to add a photo of your achievement below

MILESTONES & GOALS FOR MY SUPPORT WORKER

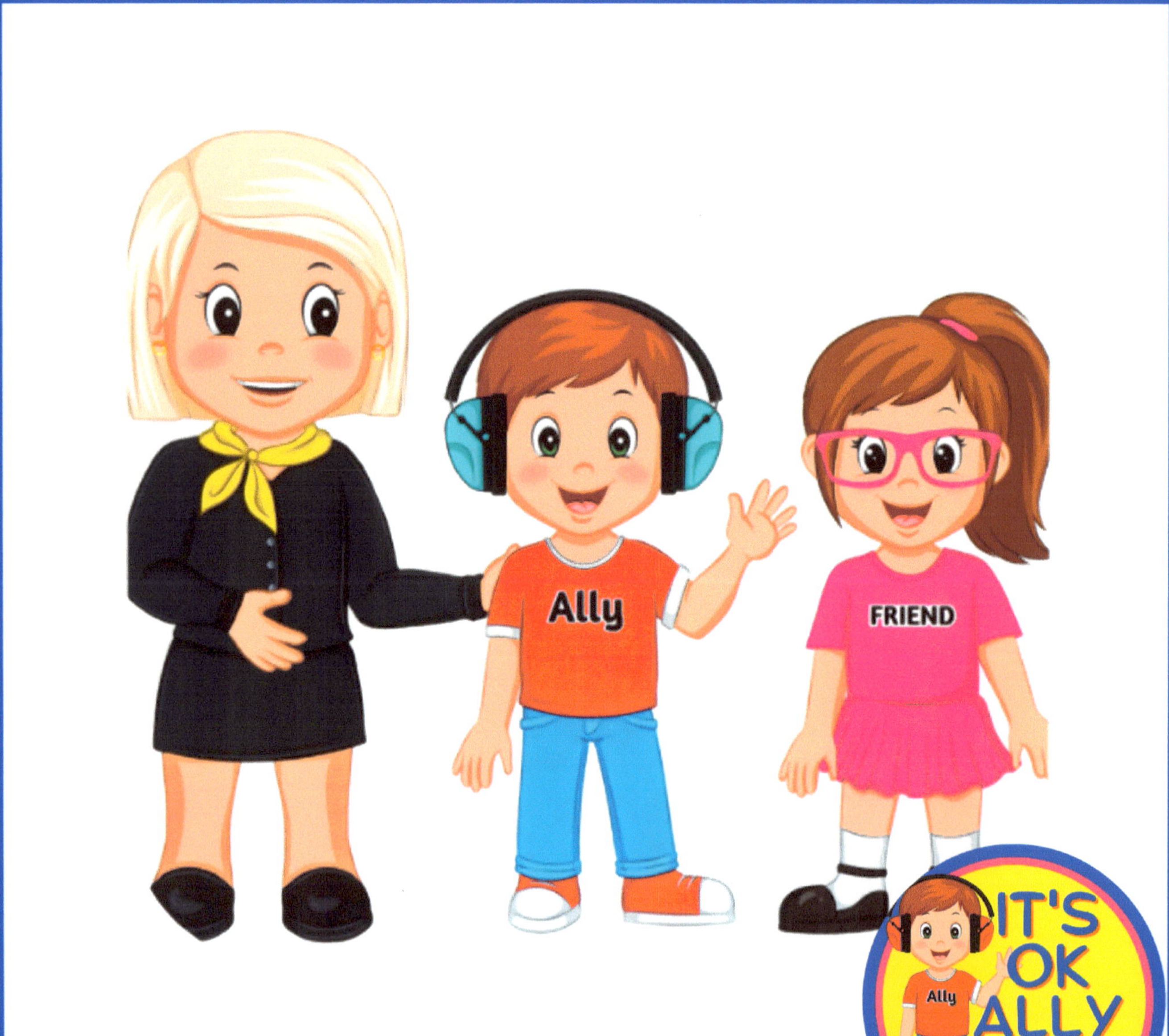

ITSOKALLY.COM

EXPENSE AND SUPPORTS TRACKER

DATE	ITEM	SPENT	REMAINS

TOTAL

NOTES	

SUPPORTS I NEED FOR MY SUPPORT WORKER

CURRENTLY MY LIFE LOOKS LIKE THIS

IN THE NEXT 12 MONTHS, I WANT TO CHANGE MY LIFE SO IT LOOKS LIKE THIS:

THE SUPPORT I NEED TO HELP ME MAKE THIS CHANGE IS:

GOALS FOR MY SUPPORT WORKER

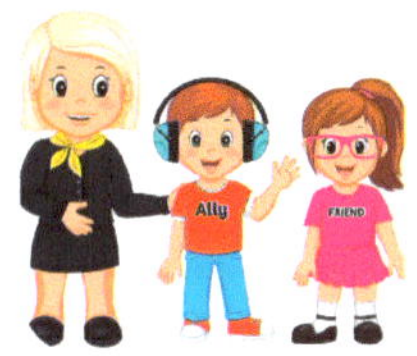

YEARLY GOAL I WOULD LIKE TO ACHIEVE

Break down your goal into 3 simple targets:

3 MONTHS	6 MONTHS	12 MONTHS
ACTiON STEPS:	ACTiON STEPS:	ACTiON STEPS:
○	○	○
○	○	○
○	○	○
○	○	○

BECAUSE OF FUNDING RECEIVED LAST YEAR, I ACHIEVED THIS GOAL IN 12 MONTHS

Achievement:
Date this occurred:
How long it took me to reach my goal:
What resources helped me reach my goal?
This new skill has helped me:

THIS IS A PHOTO OF ME ON THE DAY I ACHIEVED MY GOAL

Use the Goodnotes "Add Image" button to add a photo of your achievement below

MILESTONES & GOALS FOR MY COMMUNITY

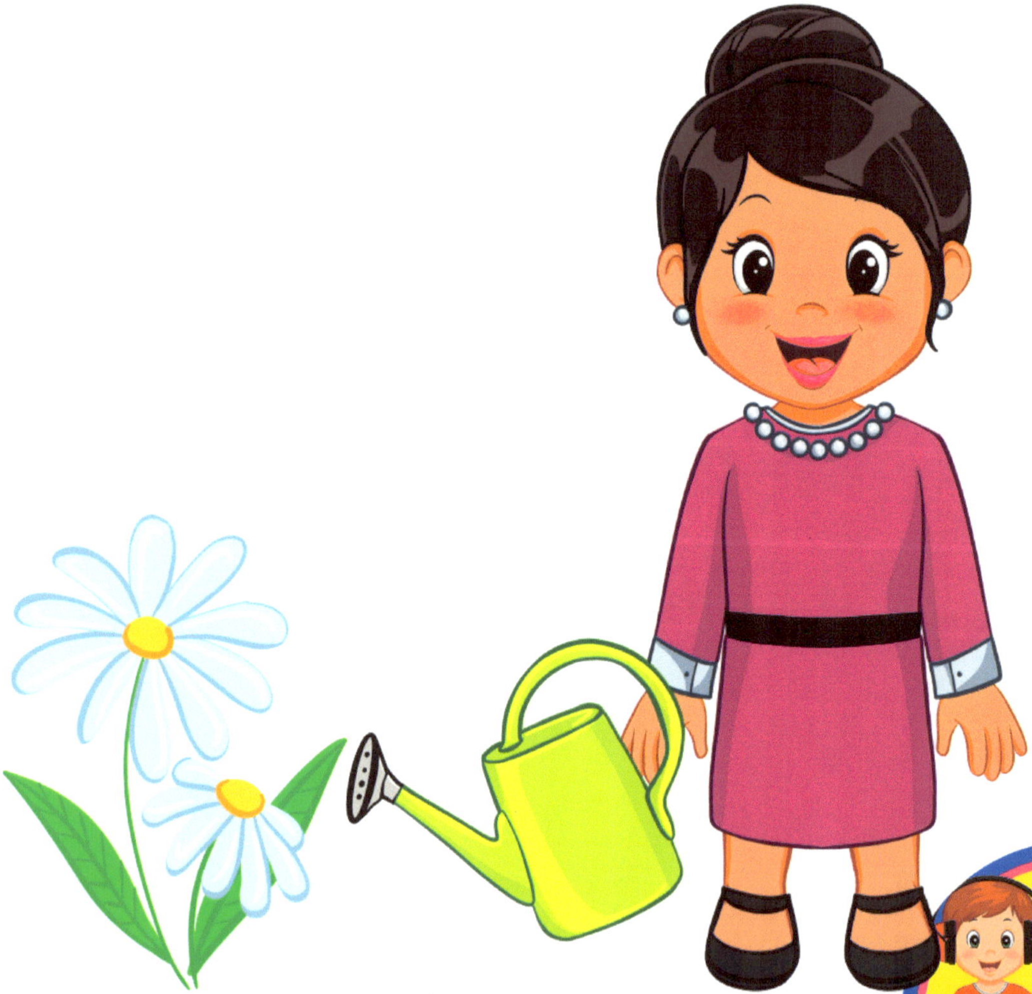

IT'S OK ALLY
CLIPART & RESOURCES FOR CHILDREN WITH SPECIAL NEEDS

ITSOKALLY.COM

EXPENSE AND SUPPORTS TRACKER

DATE	ITEM	SPENT	REMAINS

TOTAL

NOTES	

SUPPORTS I NEED FOR MY COMMUNITY

CURRENTLY MY LIFE LOOKS LIKE THIS

IN THE NEXT 12 MONTHS, I WANT TO CHANGE MY LIFE SO IT LOOKS LIKE THIS:

THE SUPPORT I NEED TO HELP ME MAKE THIS CHANGE IS:

GOALS FOR MY COMMUNiTY

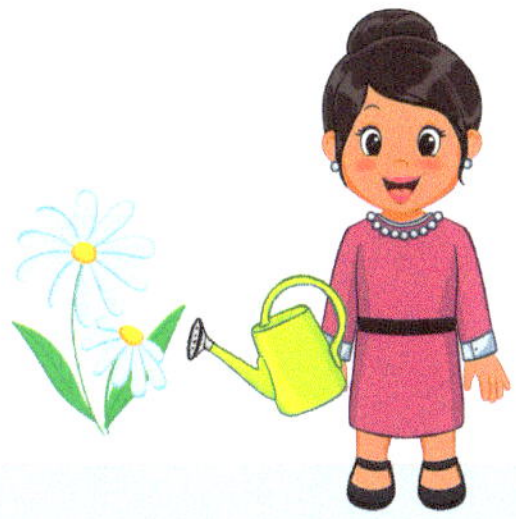

YEARLY GOAL I WOULD LIKE TO ACHIEVE

Break down your goal into 3 simple targets:

3 MONTHS	6 MONTHS	12 MONTHS
ACTiON STEPS:	ACTiON STEPS:	ACTiON STEPS:

BECAUSE OF FUNDING RECEIVED LAST YEAR, I ACHIEVED THIS GOAL IN 12 MONTHS

Achievement:
Date this occurred:
How long it took me to reach my goal:
What resources helped me reach my goal?
This new skill has helped me:

THIS IS A PHOTO OF ME ON THE DAY I ACHIEVED MY GOAL

Use the Goodnotes "Add Image" button to add a photo of your achievement below

MILESTONES & GOALS FOR MY WORK

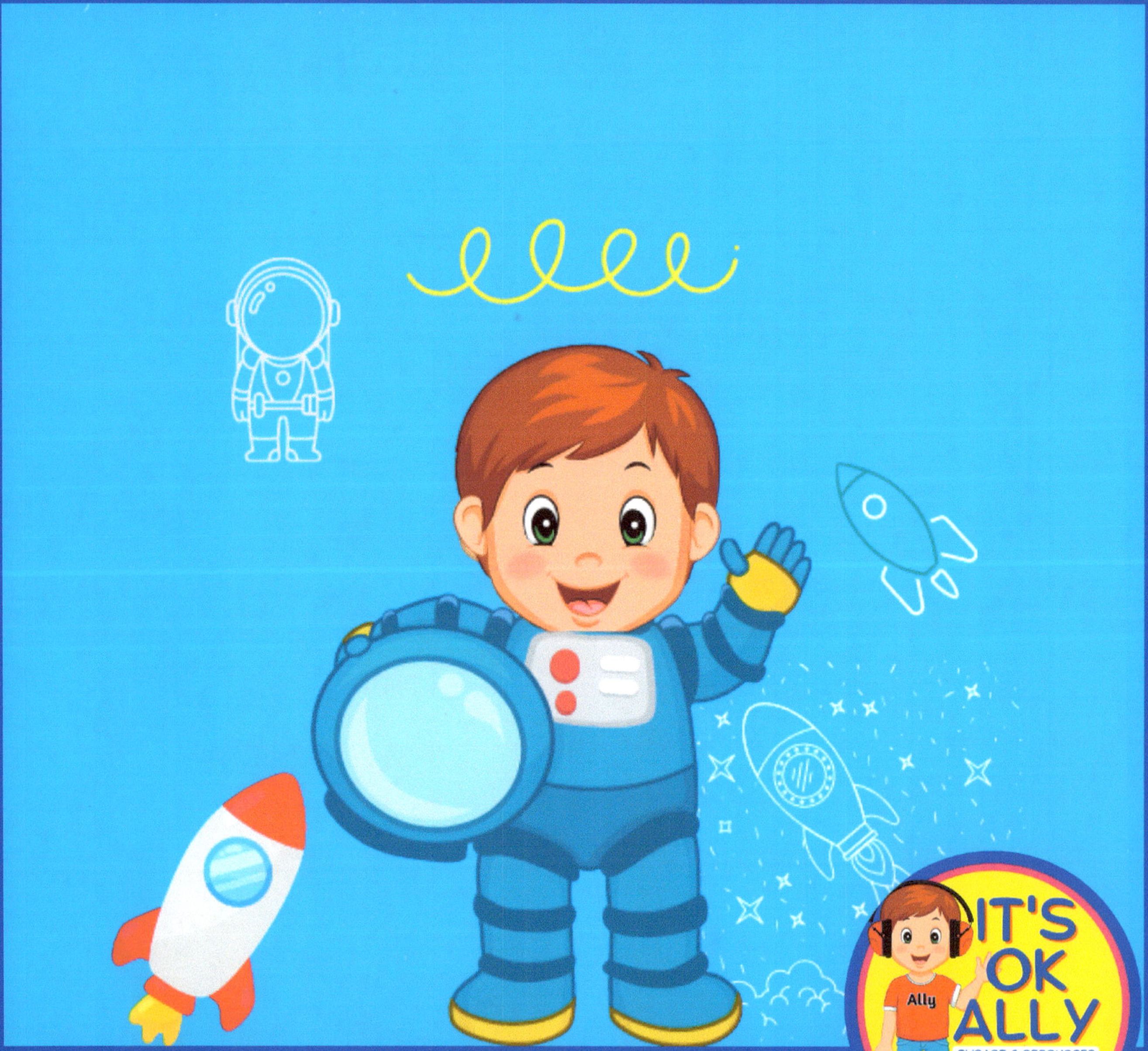

ITSOKALLY.COM

IT'S OK ALLY
CLIPART & RESOURCES FOR CHILDREN WITH SPECIAL NEEDS

EXPENSE AND SUPPORTS TRACKER

DATE	ITEM	SPENT	REMAINS

TOTAL	

NOTES	

SUPPORTS I NEED FOR MY WORK

CURRENTLY MY LIFE LOOKS LIKE THIS

IN THE NEXT 12 MONTHS, I WANT TO CHANGE MY LIFE SO IT LOOKS LIKE THIS:

THE SUPPORT I NEED TO HELP ME MAKE THIS CHANGE IS:

GOALS FOR MY WORK

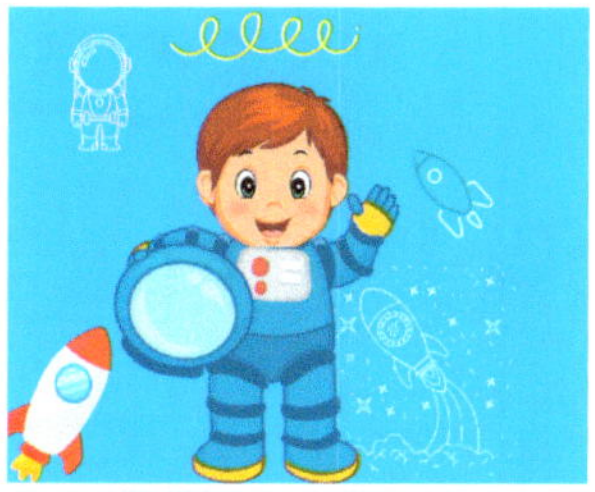

YEARLY GOAL I WOULD LIKE TO ACHIEVE

Break down your goal into 3 simple targets:

3 MONTHS	6 MONTHS	12 MONTHS

ACTION STEPS:

ACTION STEPS:

ACTION STEPS:

BECAUSE OF FUNDING RECEIVED LAST YEAR, I ACHIEVED THIS GOAL IN 12 MONTHS

IT'S OK ALLY
CLIPART & RESOURCES FOR CHILDREN WITH SPECIAL NEEDS

Achievement:
Date this occurred:
How long it took me to reach my goal:
What resources helped me reach my goal?
This new skill has helped me:

IT'S OK ALLY

CLIPART & RESOURCES FOR CHILDREN WITH SPECIAL NEEDS

THIS IS A PHOTO OF ME ON THE DAY I ACHIEVED MY GOAL

Use the Goodnotes "Add Image" button to add a photo of your achievement below

MILESTONES & GOALS FOR MY WEALTH

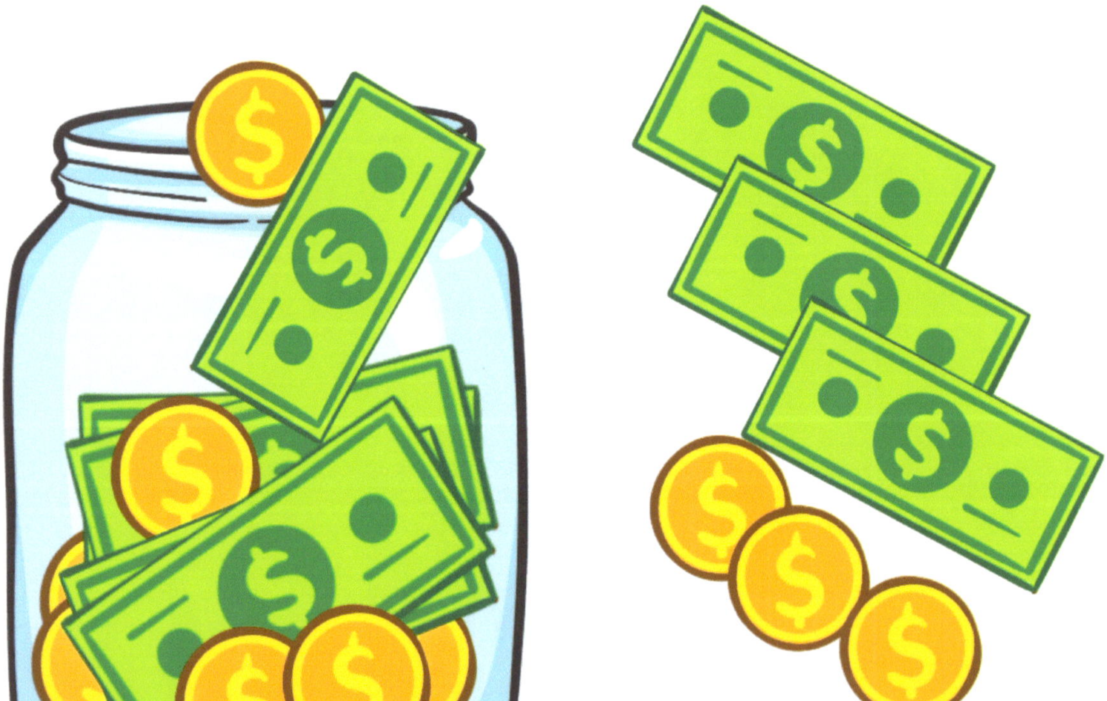

ITSOKALLY.COM

EXPENSE AND SUPPORTS TRACKER

DATE	ITEM	SPENT	REMAINS

TOTAL

NOTES	

SUPPORTS I NEED FOR MY WEALTH

CURRENTLY MY LIFE LOOKS LIKE THIS

IN THE NEXT 12 MONTHS, I WANT TO CHANGE MY LIFE SO IT LOOKS LIKE THIS:

THE SUPPORT I NEED TO HELP ME MAKE THIS CHANGE IS:

GOALS FOR MY WEALTH

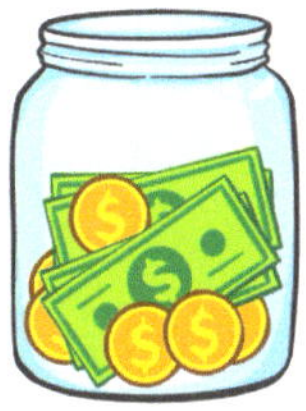

YEARLY GOAL I WOULD LIKE TO ACHIEVE

Break down your goal into 3 simple targets:

3 MONTHS	6 MONTHS	12 MONTHS
ACTION STEPS:	ACTION STEPS:	ACTION STEPS:
○	○	○
○	○	○
○	○	○
○	○	○

BECAUSE OF FUNDING RECEIVED LAST YEAR, I ACHIEVED THIS GOAL IN 12 MONTHS

Achievement:
Date this occurred:
How long it took me to reach my goal:
What resources helped me reach my goal?
This new skill has helped me:

THIS IS A PHOTO OF ME ON THE DAY I ACHIEVED MY GOAL

Use the Goodnotes "Add Image" button to add a photo of your achievement below

MILESTONES & GOALS FOR MY TRAVEL

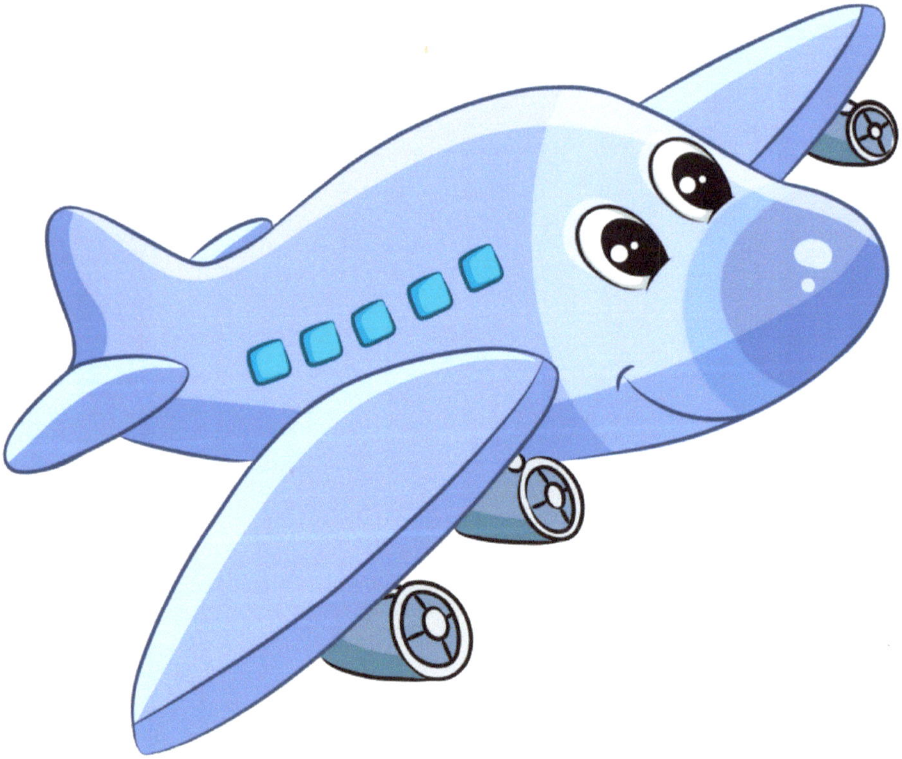

ITSOKALLY.COM

IT'S OK ALLY
CLIPART & RESOURCES FOR CHILDREN WITH SPECIAL NEEDS

EXPENSE AND SUPPORTS TRACKER

DATE	ITEM	SPENT	REMAINS

TOTAL

NOTES	

SUPPORTS I NEED FOR MY TRAVEL

CURRENTLY MY LIFE LOOKS LIKE THIS

IN THE NEXT 12 MONTHS, I WANT TO CHANGE MY LIFE SO IT LOOKS LIKE THIS:

THE SUPPORT I NEED TO HELP ME MAKE THIS CHANGE IS:

GOALS FOR MY TRAVEL

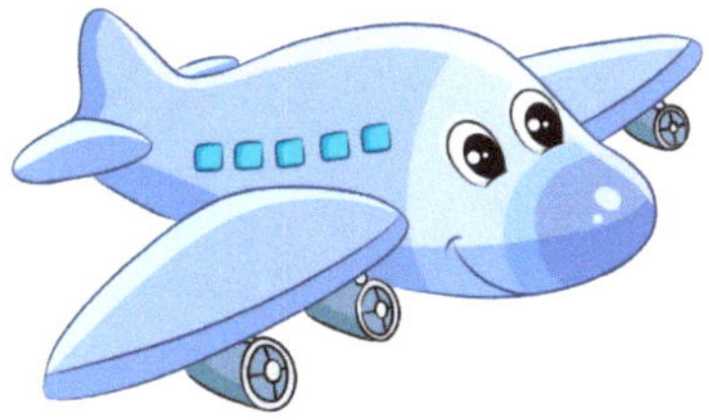

YEARLY GOAL I WOULD LIKE TO ACHIEVE

Break down your goal into 3 simple targets:

3 MONTHS	6 MONTHS	12 MONTHS
ACTION STEPS:	ACTION STEPS:	ACTION STEPS:
○	○	○
○	○	○
○	○	○
○	○	○

BECAUSE OF FUNDING RECEIVED LAST YEAR, I ACHIEVED THIS GOAL IN 12 MONTHS

Achievement:
Date this occurred:
How long it took me to reach my goal:
What resources helped me reach my goal?
This new skill has helped me:

THIS IS A PHOTO OF ME ON THE DAY I ACHIEVED MY GOAL

Use the Goodnotes "Add Image" button to add a photo of your achievement below

MILESTONES & GOALS FOR MY EXPERIENCES

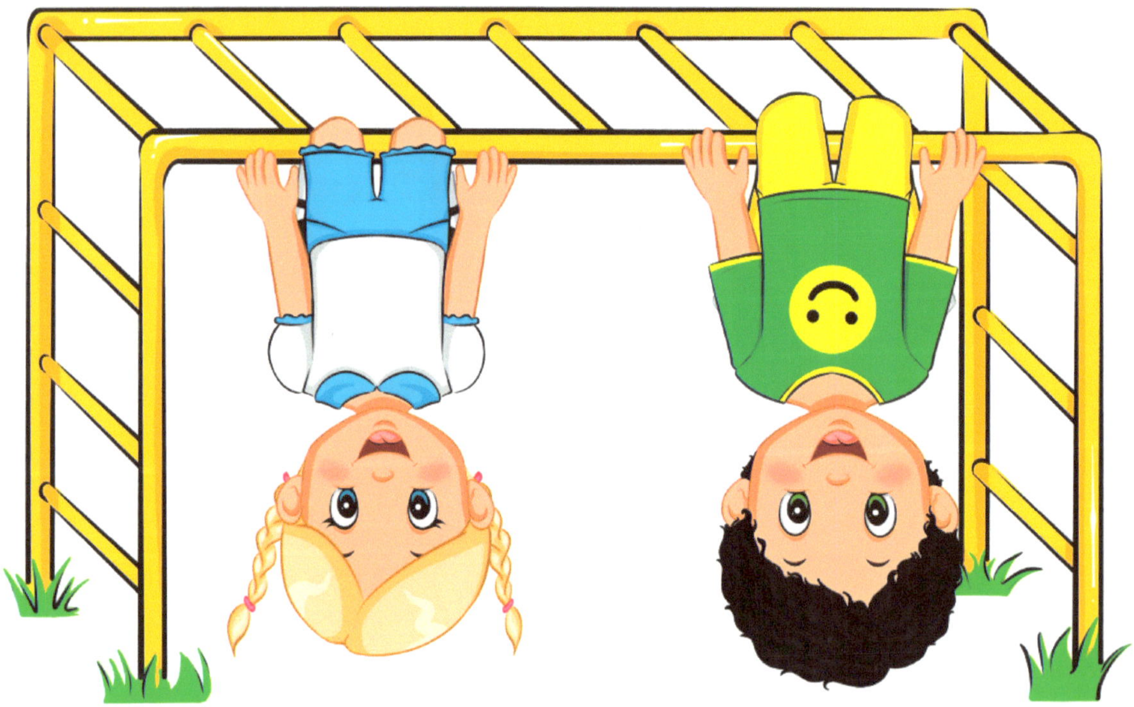

ITSOKALLY.COM

EXPENSE AND SUPPORTS TRACKER

DATE	ITEM	SPENT	REMAINS

TOTAL

NOTES	

SUPPORTS I NEED FOR MY EXPERIENCES

CURRENTLY MY LIFE LOOKS LIKE THIS

IN THE NEXT 12 MONTHS, I WANT TO CHANGE MY LIFE SO IT LOOKS LIKE THIS:

THE SUPPORT I NEED TO HELP ME MAKE THIS CHANGE IS:

GOALS FOR MY EXPERIENCES

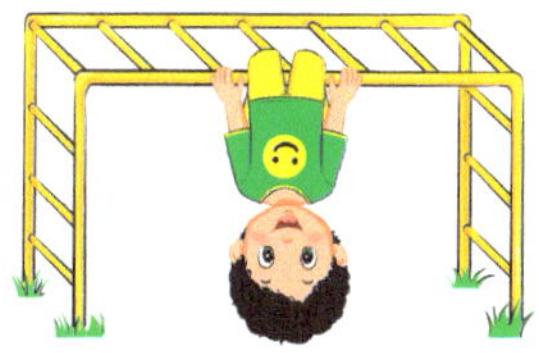

YEARLY GOAL I WOULD LIKE TO ACHIEVE

Break down your goal into 3 simple targets:

3 MONTHS	6 MONTHS	12 MONTHS
ACTION STEPS:	ACTION STEPS:	ACTION STEPS:
○	○	○
○	○	○
○	○	○
○	○	○

BECAUSE OF FUNDING RECEIVED LAST YEAR, I ACHIEVED THIS GOAL IN 12 MONTHS

Achievement:
Date this occurred:
How long it took me to reach my goal:
What resources helped me reach my goal?
This new skill has helped me:

THIS IS A PHOTO OF ME ON THE DAY I ACHIEVED MY GOAL

Use the Goodnotes "Add Image" button to add a photo of your achievement below

MILESTONES & GOALS FOR MY PERSONAL STYLE

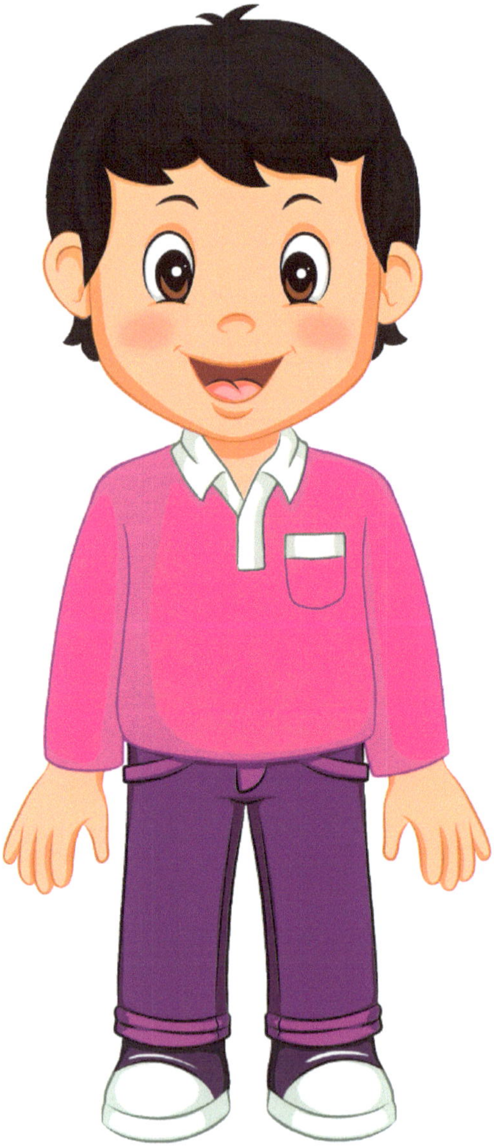

ITSOKALLY.COM

EXPENSE AND SUPPORTS TRACKER

DATE	ITEM	SPENT	REMAINS

TOTAL

NOTES	

SUPPORTS I NEED FOR MY PERSONAL STYLE

CURRENTLY MY LIFE LOOKS LIKE THIS

IN THE NEXT 12 MONTHS, I WANT TO CHANGE MY LIFE SO IT LOOKS LIKE THIS:

THE SUPPORT I NEED TO HELP ME MAKE THIS CHANGE IS:

GOALS FOR MY PERSONAL STYLE

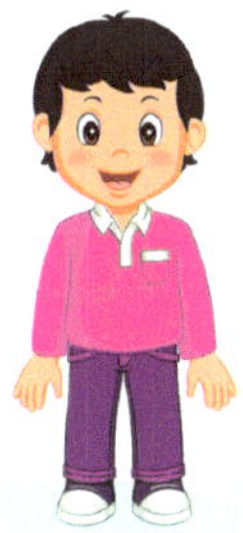

YEARLY GOAL I WOULD LIKE TO ACHIEVE

Break down your goal into 3 simple targets:

3 MONTHS	6 MONTHS	12 MONTHS

ACTION STEPS:	ACTION STEPS:	ACTION STEPS:
○	○	○
○	○	○
○	○	○
○	○	○

BECAUSE OF FUNDING RECEIVED LAST YEAR, I ACHIEVED THIS GOAL IN 12 MONTHS

Achievement:
Date this occurred:
How long it took me to reach my goal:
What resources helped me reach my goal?
This new skill has helped me:

THIS IS A PHOTO OF ME ON THE DAY I ACHIEVED MY GOAL

Use the Goodnotes "Add Image" button to add a photo of your achievement below

MILESTONES & GOALS FOR MY ASSETS

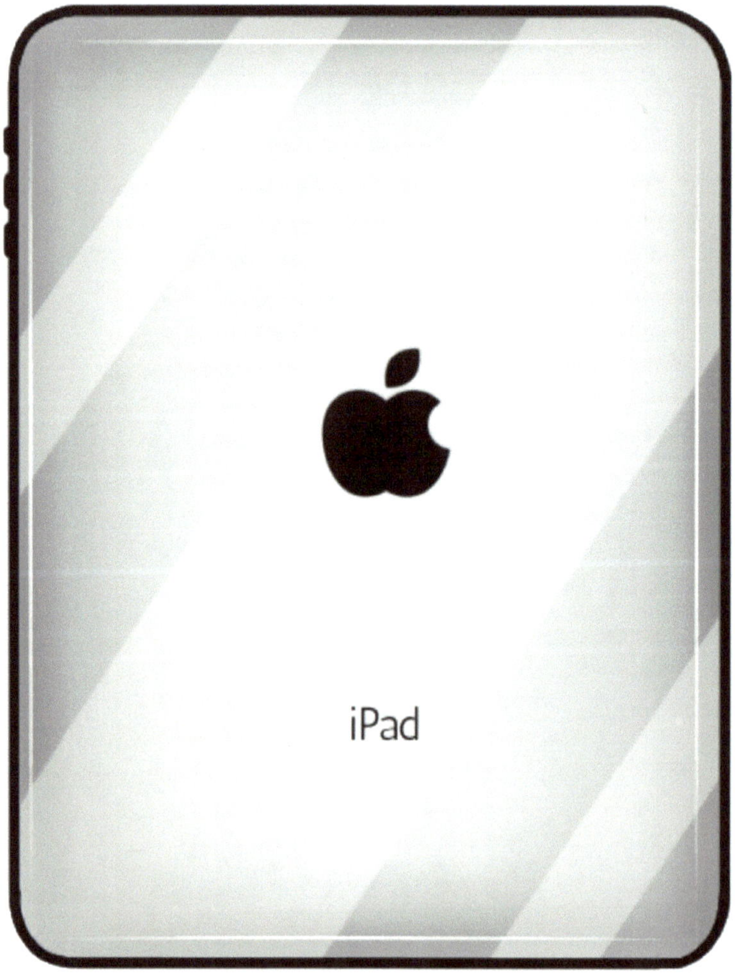

EXPENSE AND SUPPORTS TRACKER

DATE	ITEM	SPENT	REMAINS

TOTAL

NOTES	

SUPPORTS I NEED FOR MY ASSETS

CURRENTLY MY LIFE LOOKS LIKE THIS

IN THE NEXT 12 MONTHS, I WANT TO CHANGE MY LIFE SO IT LOOKS LIKE THIS:

THE SUPPORT I NEED TO HELP ME MAKE THIS CHANGE IS:

GOALS FOR MY ASSETS

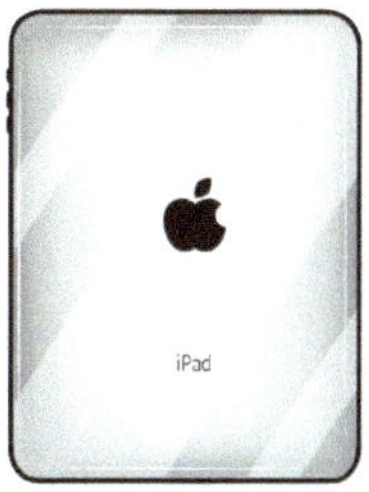

YEARLY GOAL I WOULD LIKE TO ACHIEVE

Break down your goal into 3 simple targets:

3 MONTHS

ACTION STEPS:

- ○
- ○
- ○
- ○

6 MONTHS

ACTION STEPS:

- ○
- ○
- ○
- ○

12 MONTHS

ACTION STEPS:

- ○
- ○
- ○
- ○

BECAUSE OF FUNDING RECEIVED LAST YEAR, I ACHIEVED THIS GOAL IN 12 MONTHS

IT'S OK ALLY
CLIPART & RESOURCES FOR CHILDREN WITH SPECIAL NEEDS

Achievement:
Date this occurred:
How long it took me to reach my goal:
What resources helped me reach my goal?
This new skill has helped me:

THIS IS A PHOTO OF ME ON THE DAY I ACHIEVED MY GOAL

Use the Goodnotes "Add Image" button to add a photo of your achievement below

MILESTONES & GOALS FOR MY CAR

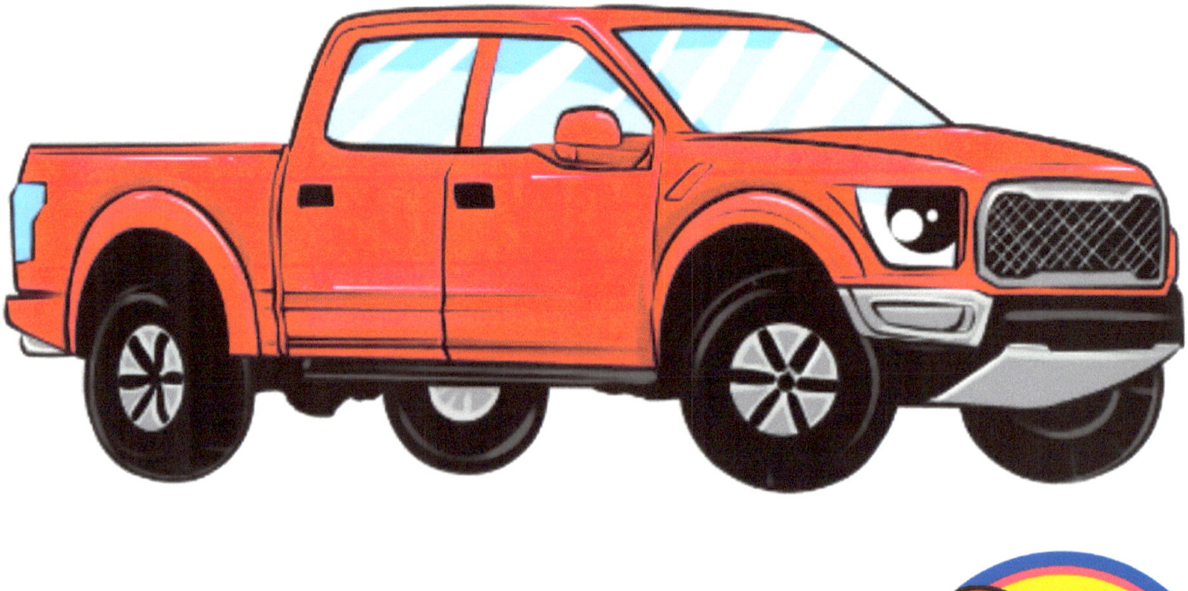

ITSOKALLY.COM

IT'S OK ALLY
CLIPART & RESOURCES FOR CHILDREN WITH SPECIAL NEEDS

EXPENSE AND SUPPORTS TRACKER

DATE	ITEM	SPENT	REMAINS

TOTAL	

NOTES	

SUPPORTS I NEED FOR MY CAR

CURRENTLY MY LIFE LOOKS LIKE THIS

IN THE NEXT 12 MONTHS, I WANT TO CHANGE MY LIFE SO IT LOOKS LIKE THIS:

THE SUPPORT I NEED TO HELP ME MAKE THIS CHANGE IS:

GOALS FOR MY CAR

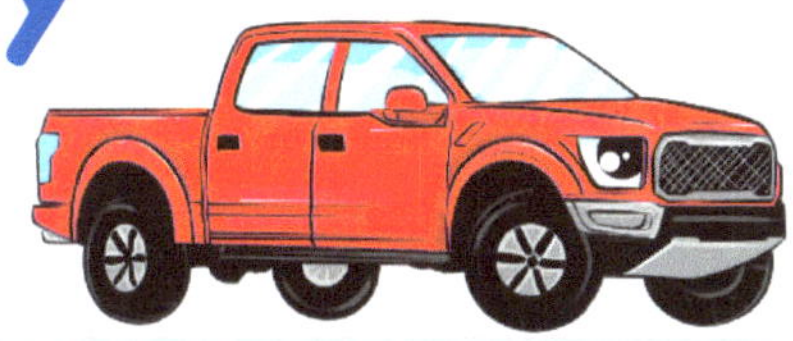

YEARLY GOAL I WOULD LIKE TO ACHIEVE

Break down your goal into 3 simple targets:

3 MONTHS	6 MONTHS	12 MONTHS
ACTION STEPS:	ACTION STEPS:	ACTION STEPS:

BECAUSE OF FUNDING RECEIVED LAST YEAR, I ACHIEVED THIS GOAL IN 12 MONTHS

Achievement:
Date this occurred:
How long it took me to reach my goal:
What resources helped me reach my goal?
This new skill has helped me:

THIS IS A PHOTO OF ME ON THE DAY I ACHIEVED MY GOAL

Use the Goodnotes "Add Image" button to add a photo of your achievement below

MILESTONES & GOALS FOR MY PET

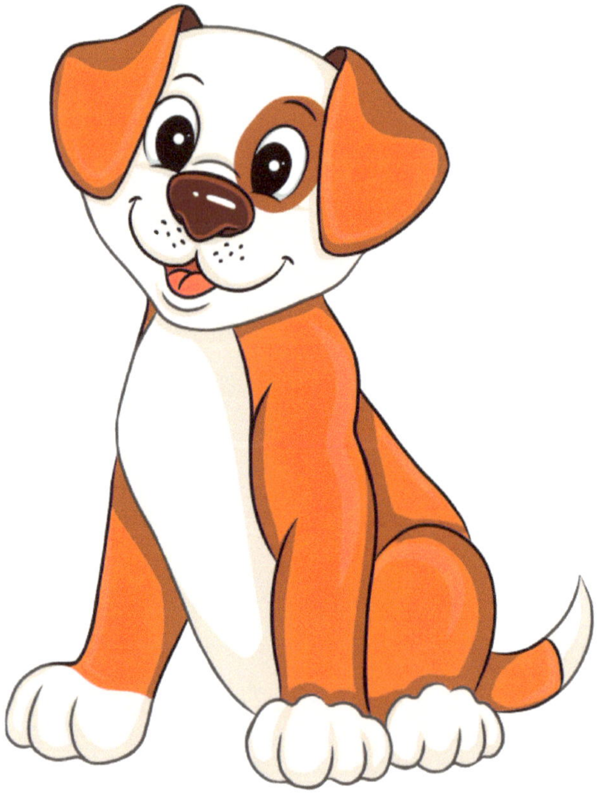

ITSOKALLY.COM

EXPENSE AND SUPPORTS TRACKER

DATE	ITEM	SPENT	REMAINS

TOTAL

NOTES	

SUPPORTS I NEED FOR MY PET

CURRENTLY MY LIFE LOOKS LIKE THIS

IN THE NEXT 12 MONTHS, I WANT TO CHANGE MY LIFE SO IT LOOKS LIKE THIS:

THE SUPPORT I NEED TO HELP ME MAKE THIS CHANGE IS:

GOALS FOR MY PET

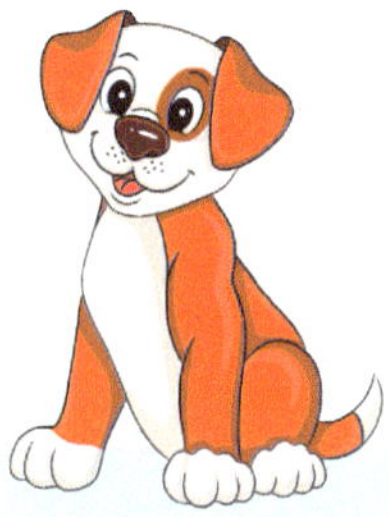

YEARLY GOAL I WOULD LIKE TO ACHIEVE

Break down your goal into 3 simple targets:

3 MONTHS	6 MONTHS	12 MONTHS
ACTION STEPS:	ACTION STEPS:	ACTION STEPS:

BECAUSE OF FUNDING RECEIVED LAST YEAR, I ACHIEVED THIS GOAL IN 12 MONTHS

Achievement:
Date this occurred:
How long it took me to reach my goal:
What resources helped me reach my goal?
This new skill has helped me:

THIS IS A PHOTO OF ME ON THE DAY I ACHIEVED MY GOAL

Use the Goodnotes "Add Image" button to add a photo of your achievement below

MILESTONES & GOALS FOR MY DAILY ACTIVITIES

ITSOKALLY.COM

EXPENSE AND SUPPORTS TRACKER

DATE	ITEM	SPENT	REMAINS

TOTAL

NOTES	

SUPPORTS I NEED FOR MY DAILY ACTIVITIES

CURRENTLY MY LIFE LOOKS LIKE THIS

IN THE NEXT 12 MONTHS, I WANT TO CHANGE MY LIFE SO IT LOOKS LIKE THIS:

THE SUPPORT I NEED TO HELP ME MAKE THIS CHANGE IS:

GOALS FOR MY DAILY ACTIVITIES

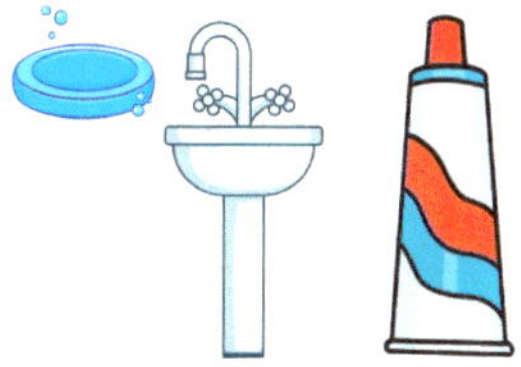

YEARLY GOAL I WOULD LIKE TO ACHIEVE

Break down your goal into 3 simple targets:

3 MONTHS	6 MONTHS	12 MONTHS
ACTION STEPS:	ACTION STEPS:	ACTION STEPS:
○	○	○
○	○	○
○	○	○
○	○	○

BECAUSE OF FUNDING RECEIVED LAST YEAR, I ACHIEVED THIS GOAL IN 12 MONTHS

Achievement:
Date this occurred:
How long it took me to reach my goal:
What resources helped me reach my goal?
This new skill has helped me:

THIS IS A PHOTO OF ME ON THE DAY I ACHIEVED MY GOAL

Use the Goodnotes "Add Image" button to add a photo of your achievement below

MILESTONES & GOALS FOR MY WEEKEND ACTIVITIES

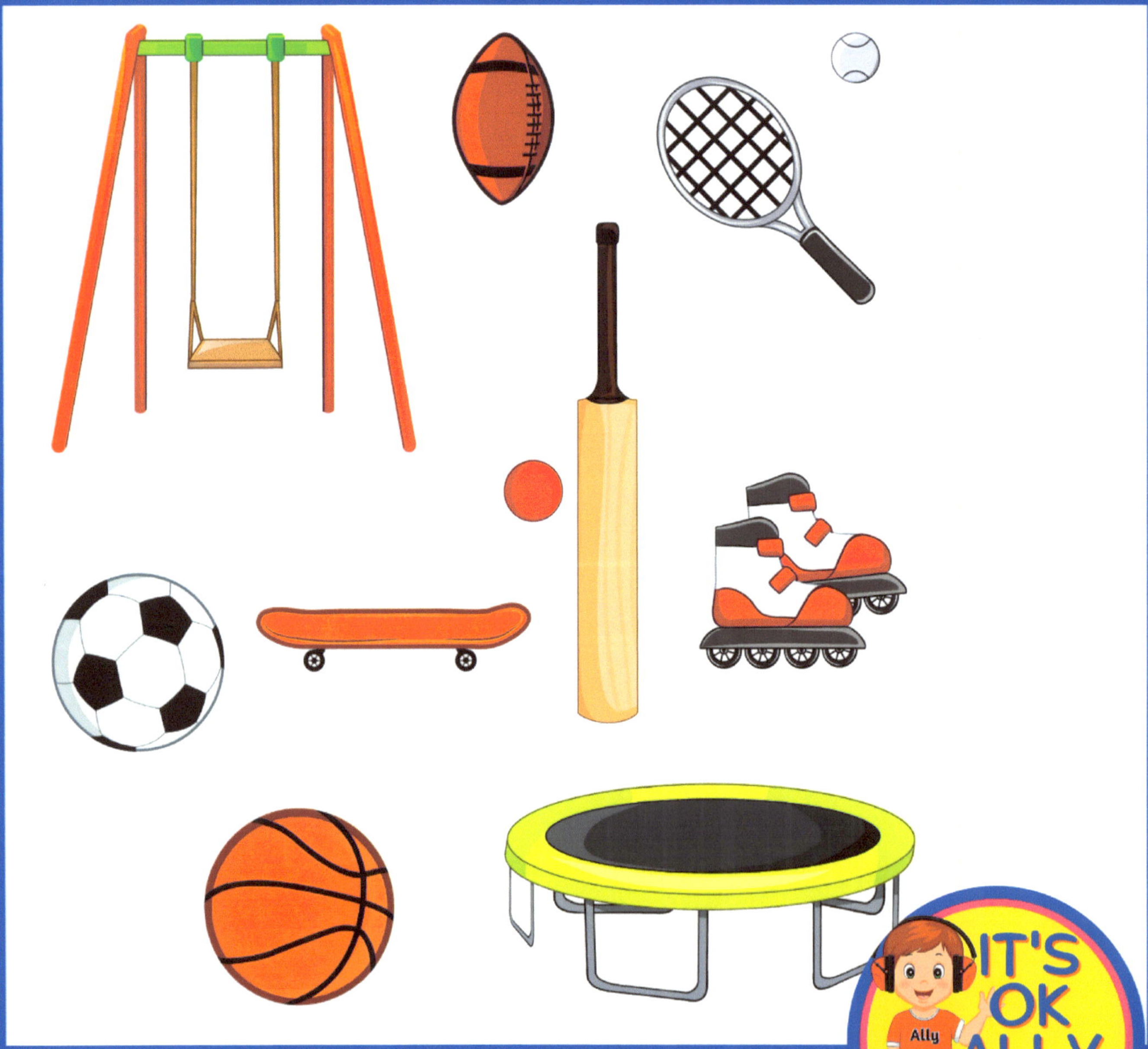

ITSOKALLY.COM

EXPENSE AND SUPPORTS TRACKER

DATE	ITEM	SPENT	REMAINS

TOTAL	

NOTES	

SUPPORTS I NEED FOR MY WEEKEND ACTIVITIES

CURRENTLY MY LIFE LOOKS LIKE THIS

IN THE NEXT 12 MONTHS, I WANT TO CHANGE MY LIFE SO IT LOOKS LIKE THIS:

THE SUPPORT I NEED TO HELP ME MAKE THIS CHANGE IS:

GOALS FOR MY WEEKEND ACTIVITIES

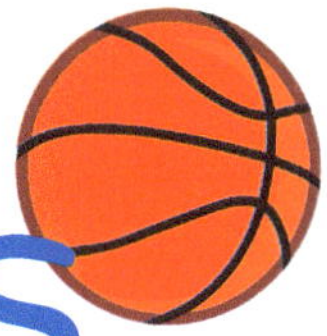

YEARLY GOAL I WOULD LIKE TO ACHIEVE

Break down your goal into 3 simple targets:

3 MONTHS	6 MONTHS	12 MONTHS
ACTION STEPS:	ACTION STEPS:	ACTION STEPS:
○	○	○
○	○	○
○	○	○
○	○	○

BECAUSE OF FUNDING RECEIVED LAST YEAR, I ACHIEVED THIS GOAL IN 12 MONTHS

Achievement:
Date this occurred:
How long it took me to reach my goal:
What resources helped me reach my goal?
This new skill has helped me:

THIS IS A PHOTO OF ME ON THE DAY I ACHIEVED MY GOAL

Use the Goodnotes "Add Image" button to add a photo of your achievement below

MILESTONES & GOALS FOR MY CREATIVE ACTIVITIES

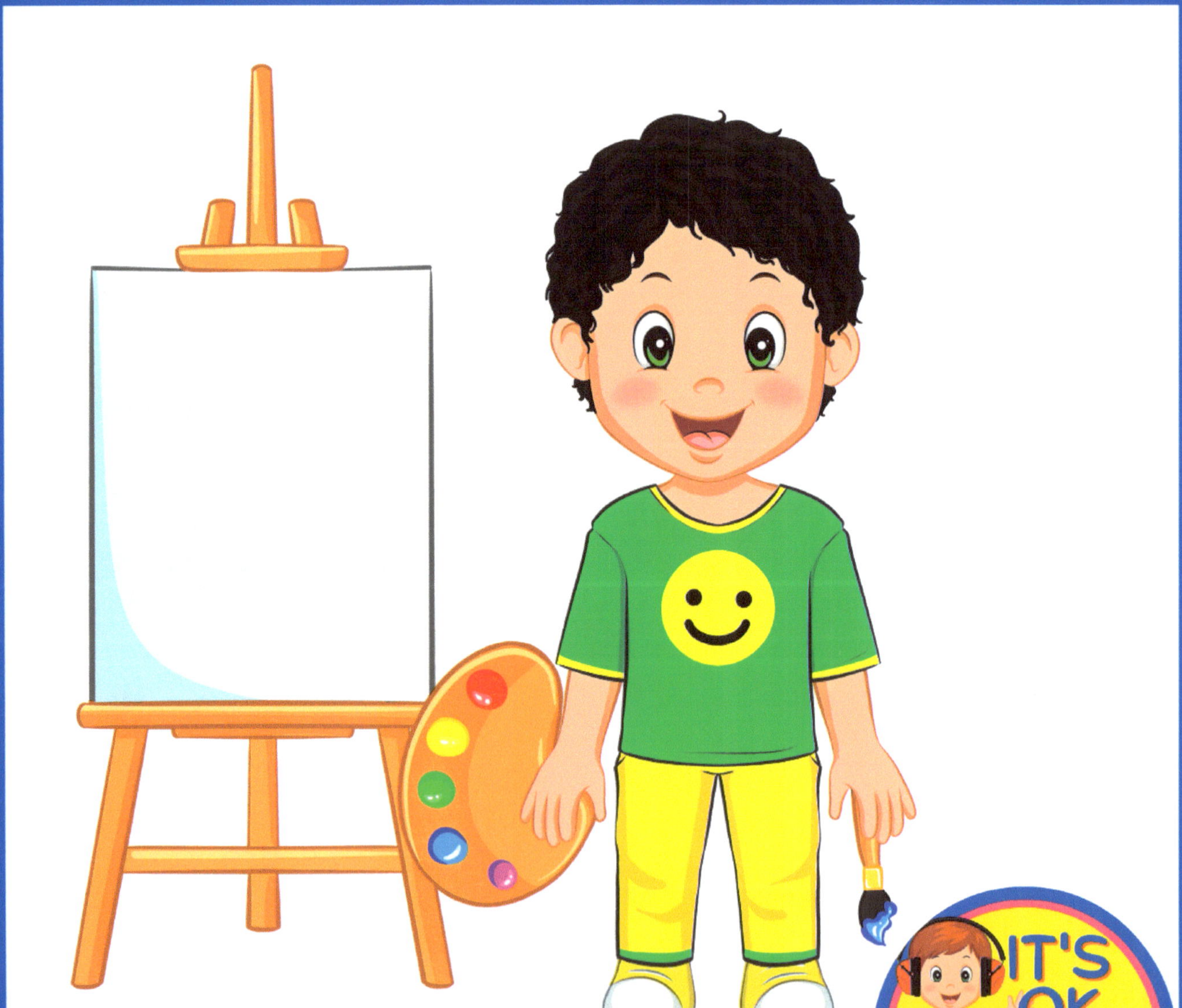

IT'S OK ALLY
CLIPART & RESOURCES FOR CHILDREN WITH SPECIAL NEEDS

ITSOKALLY.COM

EXPENSE AND SUPPORTS TRACKER

DATE	ITEM	SPENT	REMAINS

TOTAL

NOTES	

SUPPORTS I NEED FOR MY CREATIVE ACTIVITIES

CURRENTLY MY LIFE LOOKS LIKE THIS

IN THE NEXT 12 MONTHS, I WANT TO CHANGE MY LIFE SO IT LOOKS LIKE THIS:

THE SUPPORT I NEED TO HELP ME MAKE THIS CHANGE IS:

GOALS FOR MY CREATIVE ACTIVITIES

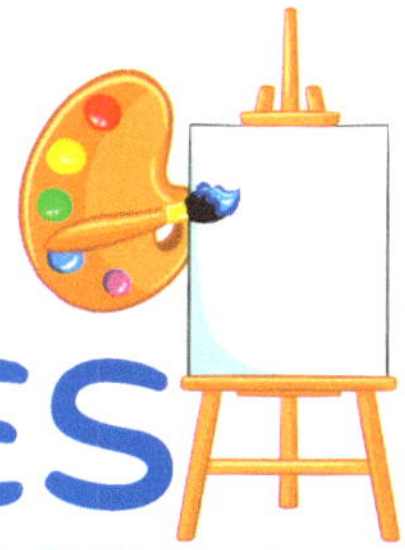

YEARLY GOAL I WOULD LIKE TO ACHIEVE

Break down your goal into 3 simple targets:

3 MONTHS	6 MONTHS	12 MONTHS
ACTION STEPS:	ACTION STEPS:	ACTION STEPS:
○	○	○
○	○	○
○	○	○
○	○	○

BECAUSE OF FUNDING RECEIVED LAST YEAR, I ACHIEVED THIS GOAL IN 12 MONTHS

Achievement:
Date this occurred:
How long it took me to reach my goal:
What resources helped me reach my goal?
This new skill has helped me:

THIS IS A PHOTO OF ME ON THE DAY I ACHIEVED MY GOAL

Use the Goodnotes "Add Image" button to add a photo of your achievement below

MILESTONES & GOALS FOR MY SPECIAL ACTIVITIES

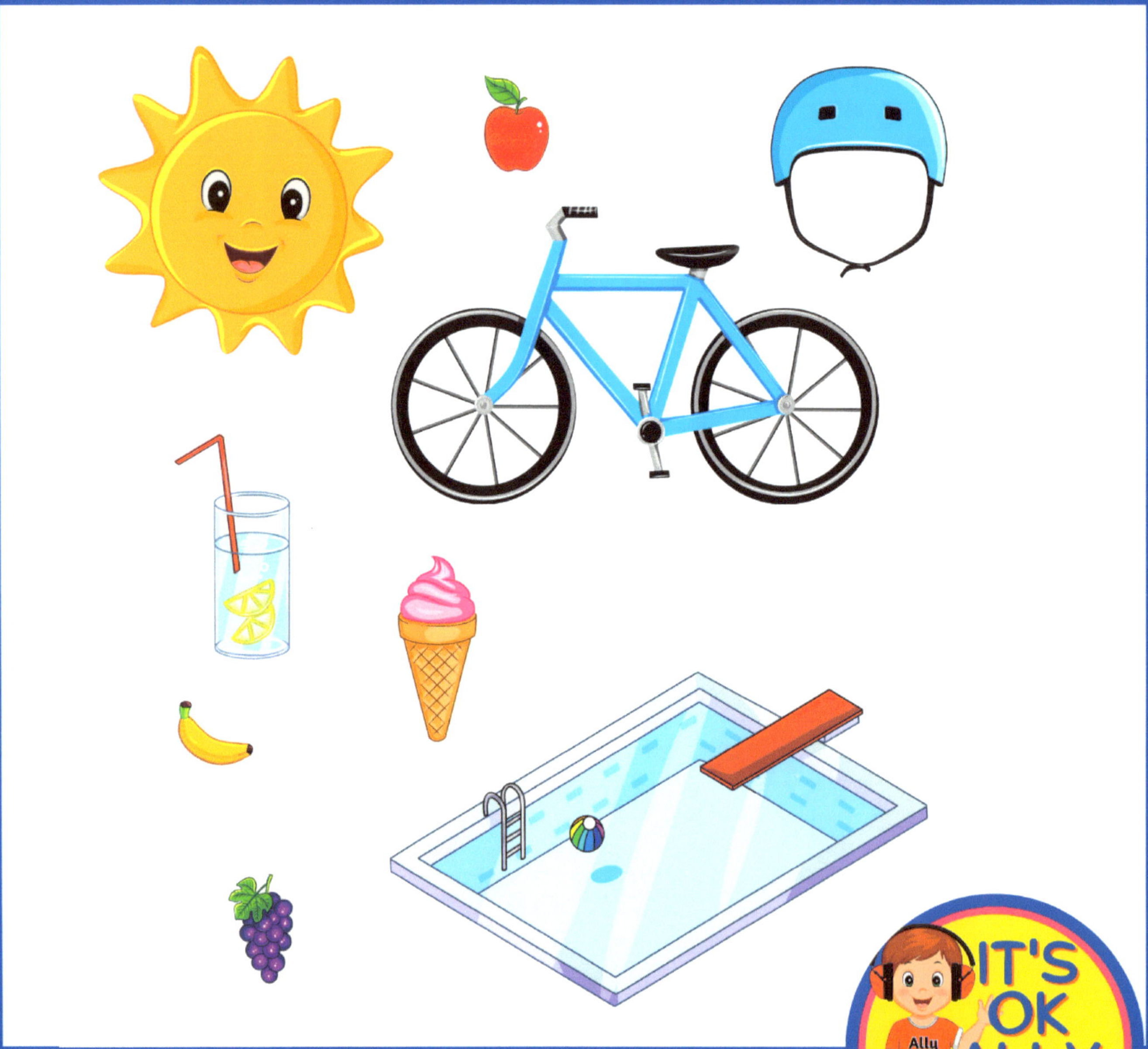

IT'S OK ALLY
CLIPART & RESOURCES FOR CHILDREN WITH SPECIAL NEEDS

ITSOKALLY.COM

EXPENSE AND SUPPORTS TRACKER

DATE	ITEM	SPENT	REMAINS

TOTAL

NOTES	

SUPPORTS I NEED FOR MY SPECIAL ACTIVITIES

CURRENTLY MY LIFE LOOKS LIKE THIS

IN THE NEXT 12 MONTHS, I WANT TO CHANGE MY LIFE SO IT LOOKS LIKE THIS:

THE SUPPORT I NEED TO HELP ME MAKE THIS CHANGE IS:

GOALS FOR MY SPECIAL ACTIVITIE

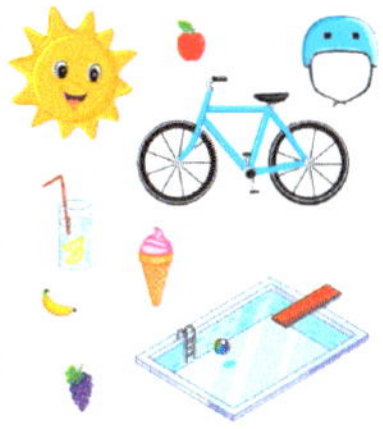

YEARLY GOAL I WOULD LIKE TO ACHIEVE

Break down your goal into 3 simple targets:

3 MONTHS

ACTION STEPS:

- ○
- ○
- ○
- ○

6 MONTHS

ACTION STEPS:

- ○
- ○
- ○
- ○

12 MONTHS

ACTION STEPS:

- ○
- ○
- ○
- ○

BECAUSE OF FUNDING RECEIVED LAST YEAR, I ACHIEVED THIS GOAL IN 12 MONTHS

Achievement:
Date this occurred:
How long it took me to reach my goal:
What resources helped me reach my goal?
This new skill has helped me:

THIS IS A PHOTO OF ME ON THE DAY I ACHIEVED MY GOAL

Use the Goodnotes "Add Image" button to add a photo of your achievement below

MILESTONES & GOALS FOR MY LEARNING

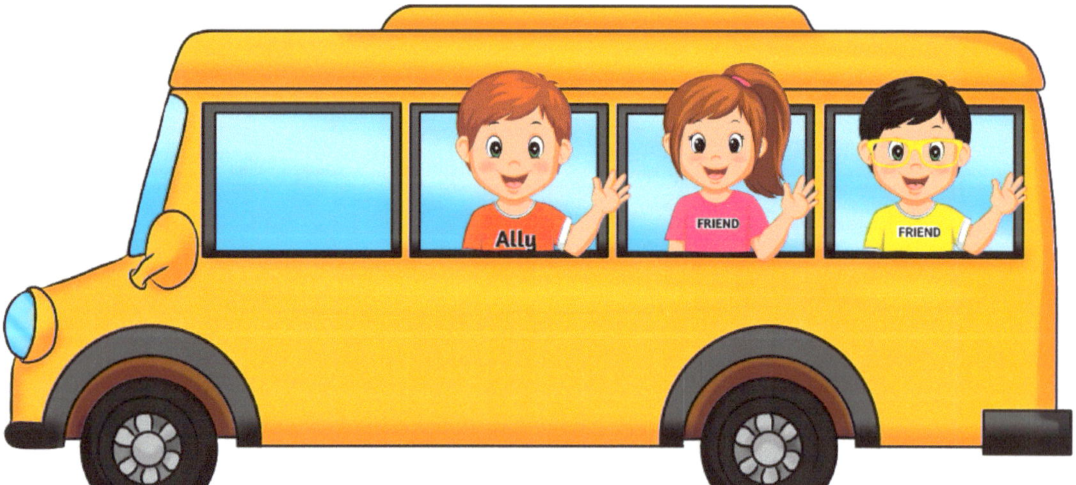

IT'S OK ALLY
CLIPART & RESOURCES FOR CHILDREN WITH SPECIAL NEEDS

ITSOKALLY.COM

EXPENSE AND SUPPORTS TRACKER

DATE	ITEM	SPENT	REMAINS

TOTAL

NOTES	

SUPPORTS I NEED FOR MY LEARNING

CURRENTLY MY LIFE LOOKS LIKE THIS

IN THE NEXT 12 MONTHS, I WANT TO CHANGE MY LIFE SO IT LOOKS LIKE THIS:

THE SUPPORT I NEED TO HELP ME MAKE THIS CHANGE IS:

GOALS FOR MY LEARNING

YEARLY GOAL I WOULD LIKE TO ACHIEVE

Break down your goal into 3 simple targets:

3 MONTHS	6 MONTHS	12 MONTHS
ACTION STEPS:	ACTION STEPS:	ACTION STEPS:
○	○	○
○	○	○
○	○	○
○	○	○

BECAUSE OF FUNDING RECEIVED LAST YEAR, I ACHIEVED THIS GOAL IN 12 MONTHS

Achievement:
Date this occurred:
How long it took me to reach my goal:
What resources helped me reach my goal?
This new skill has helped me:

THIS IS A PHOTO OF ME ON THE DAY I ACHIEVED MY GOAL

Use the Goodnotes "Add Image" button to add a photo of your achievement below

MILESTONES & GOALS FOR MY SPIRITUALITY

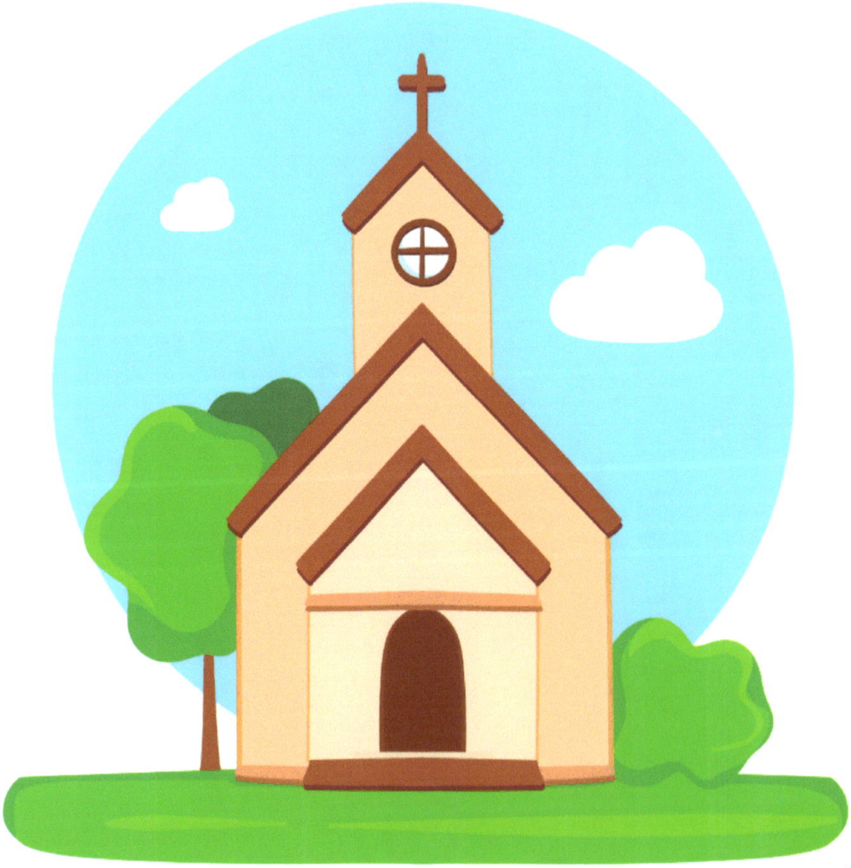

ITSOKALLY.COM

IT'S OK ALLY
CLIPART & RESOURCES FOR CHILDREN WITH SPECIAL NEEDS

EXPENSE AND SUPPORTS TRACKER

DATE	ITEM	SPENT	REMAINS

TOTAL

NOTES	

SUPPORTS I NEED FOR MY SPIRITUALITY

CURRENTLY MY LIFE LOOKS LIKE THIS

IN THE NEXT 12 MONTHS, I WANT TO CHANGE MY LIFE SO IT LOOKS LIKE THIS:

THE SUPPORT I NEED TO HELP ME MAKE THIS CHANGE IS:

GOALS FOR MY SPIRITUALITY

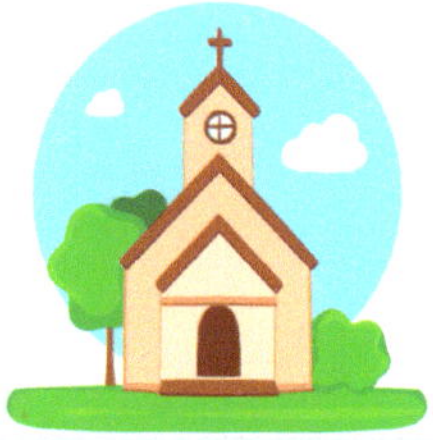

YEARLY GOAL I WOULD LIKE TO ACHIEVE

Break down your goal into 3 simple targets:

3 MONTHS	6 MONTHS	12 MONTHS
ACTION STEPS:	ACTION STEPS:	ACTION STEPS:

BECAUSE OF FUNDING RECEIVED LAST YEAR, I ACHIEVED THIS GOAL IN 12 MONTHS

Achievement:
Date this occurred:
How long it took me to reach my goal:
What resources helped me reach my goal?
This new skill has helped me:

THIS IS A PHOTO OF ME ON THE DAY I ACHIEVED MY GOAL

Use the Goodnotes "Add Image" button to add a photo of your achievement below

MILESTONES & GOALS FOR MY CHARITY

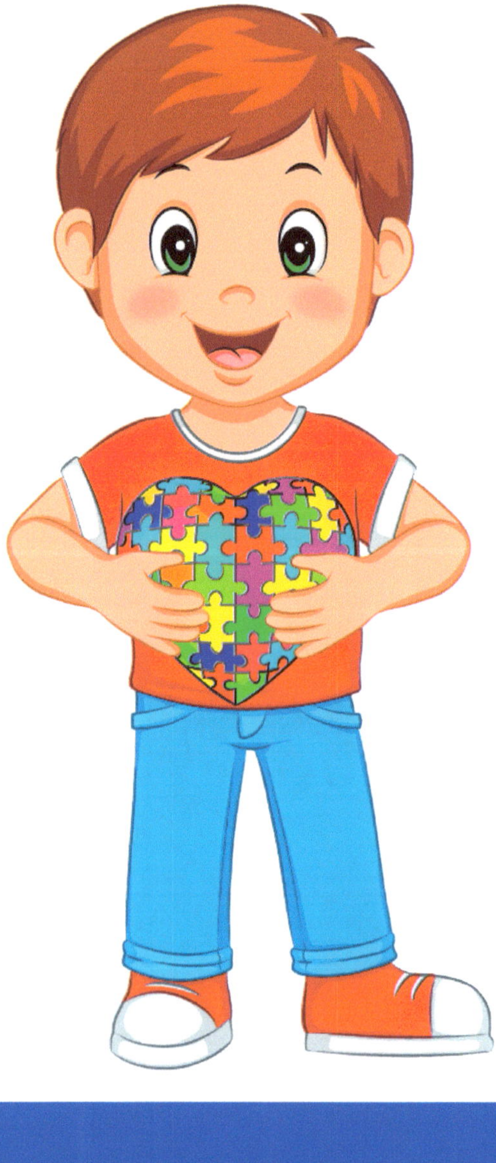

ITSOKALLY.COM

EXPENSE AND SUPPORTS TRACKER

DATE	ITEM	SPENT	REMAINS

TOTAL

NOTES	

SUPPORTS I NEED FOR MY CHARITY

CURRENTLY MY LIFE LOOKS LIKE THIS

IN THE NEXT 12 MONTHS, I WANT TO CHANGE MY LIFE SO IT LOOKS LIKE THIS:

THE SUPPORT I NEED TO HELP ME MAKE THIS CHANGE IS:

GOALS FOR MY CHARITY

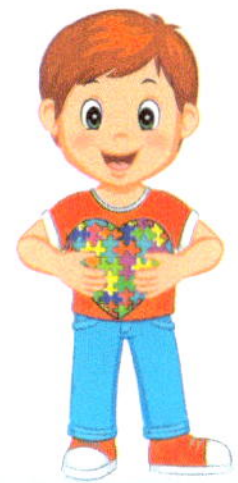

YEARLY GOAL I WOULD LIKE TO ACHIEVE

Break down your goal into 3 simple targets:

3 MONTHS	6 MONTHS	12 MONTHS
ACTION STEPS:	ACTION STEPS:	ACTION STEPS:

BECAUSE OF FUNDING RECEIVED LAST YEAR, I ACHIEVED THIS GOAL IN 12 MONTHS

IT'S OK ALLY
CLIPART & RESOURCES FOR CHILDREN WITH SPECIAL NEEDS

Achievement:
Date this occurred:
How long it took me to reach my goal:
What resources helped me reach my goal?
This new skill has helped me:

THIS IS A PHOTO OF ME ON THE DAY I ACHIEVED MY GOAL

Use the Goodnotes "Add Image" button to add a photo of your achievement below

MILESTONES & GOALS FOR MY ENVIRONMENT

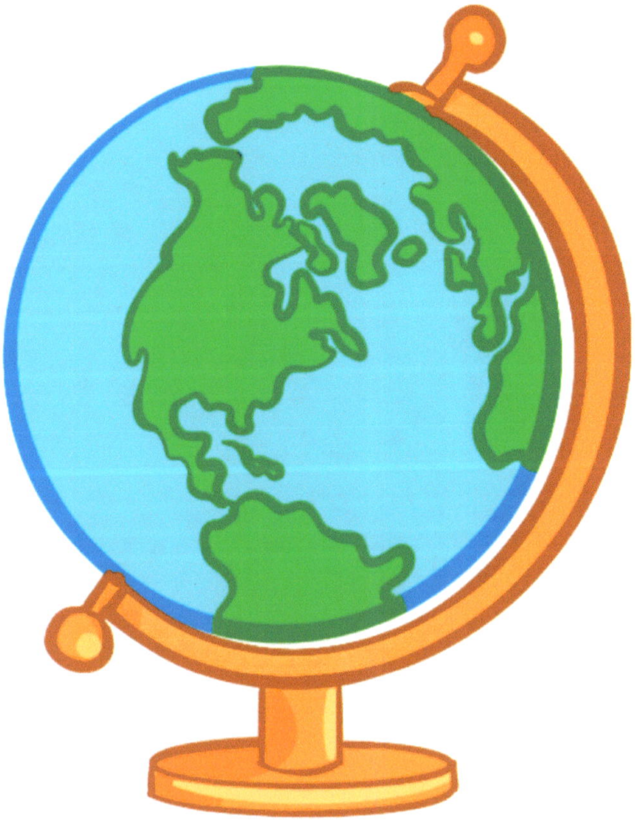

EXPENSE AND SUPPORTS TRACKER

DATE	ITEM	SPENT	REMAINS

TOTAL

NOTES	

SUPPORTS I NEED FOR MY ENVIRONMENT

CURRENTLY MY LIFE LOOKS LIKE THIS

IN THE NEXT 12 MONTHS, I WANT TO CHANGE MY LIFE SO IT LOOKS LIKE THIS:

THE SUPPORT I NEED TO HELP ME MAKE THIS CHANGE IS:

GOALS FOR MY ENVIRONMENT

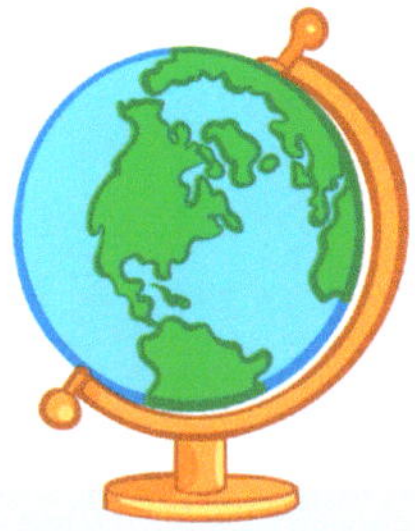

YEARLY GOAL I WOULD LIKE TO ACHIEVE

Break down your goal into 3 simple targets:

3 MONTHS	6 MONTHS	12 MONTHS
ACTION STEPS:	ACTION STEPS:	ACTION STEPS:
○	○	○
○	○	○
○	○	○
○	○	○

BECAUSE OF FUNDING RECEIVED LAST YEAR, I ACHIEVED THIS GOAL IN 12 MONTHS

Achievement:
Date this occurred:
How long it took me to reach my goal:
What resources helped me reach my goal?
This new skill has helped me:

THIS IS A PHOTO OF ME ON THE DAY I ACHIEVED MY GOAL

Use the Goodnotes "Add Image" button to add a photo of your achievement below

MILESTONES & GOALS FOR MY HOLIDAY HOME

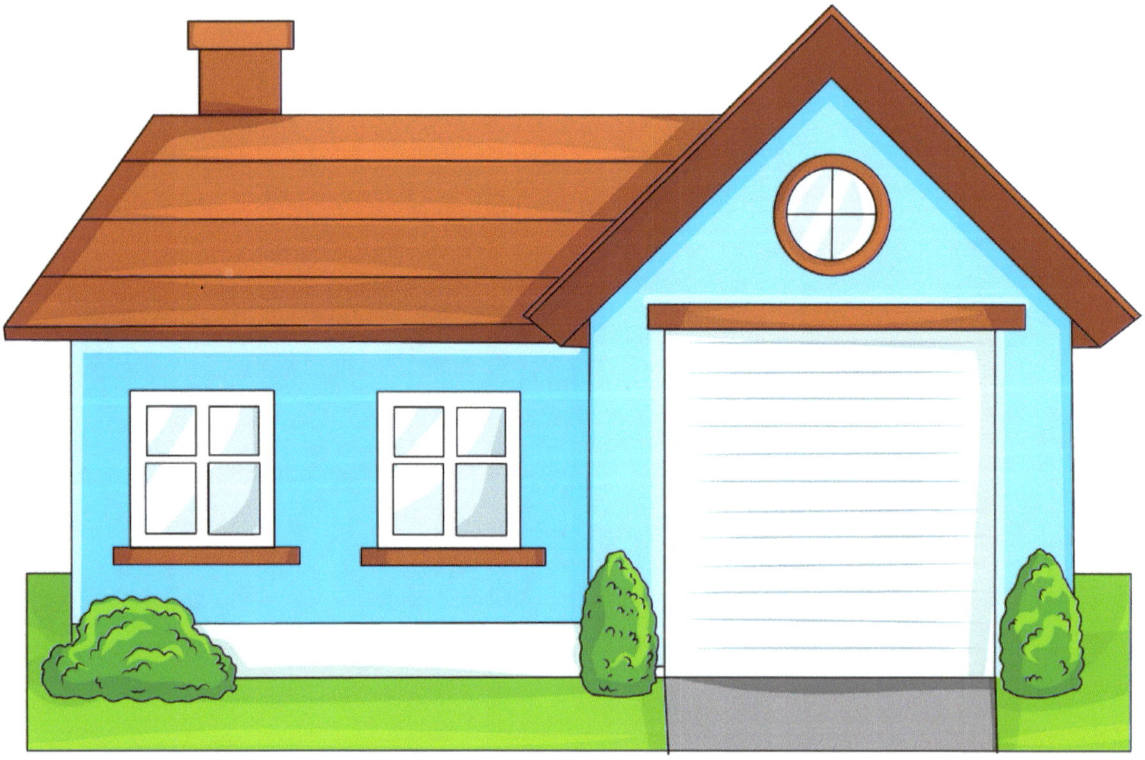

IT'S OK ALLY
CLIPART & RESOURCES FOR CHILDREN WITH SPECIAL NEEDS

EXPENSE AND SUPPORTS TRACKER

DATE	ITEM	SPENT	REMAINS

TOTAL

NOTES	

SUPPORTS I NEED FOR MY HOLIDAY HOME

CURRENTLY MY LIFE LOOKS LIKE THIS

IN THE NEXT 12 MONTHS, I WANT TO CHANGE MY LIFE SO IT LOOKS LIKE THIS:

THE SUPPORT I NEED TO HELP ME MAKE THIS CHANGE IS:

GOALS FOR MY HOLIDAY HOME

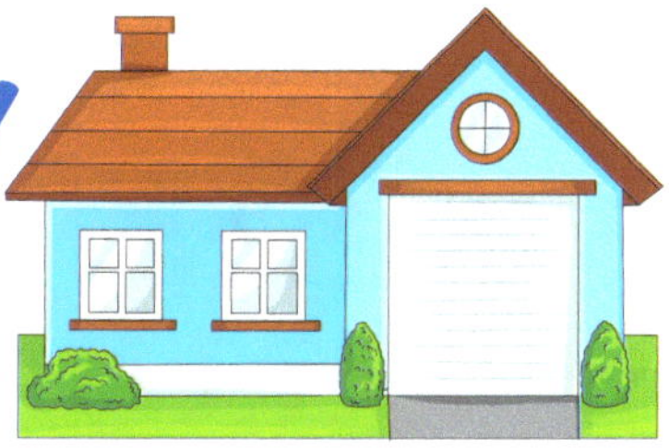

YEARLY GOAL I WOULD LIKE TO ACHIEVE

Break down your goal into 3 simple targets:

3 MONTHS	6 MONTHS	12 MONTHS

ACTION STEPS:	ACTION STEPS:	ACTION STEPS:
○	○	○
○	○	○
○	○	○
○	○	○

BECAUSE OF FUNDING RECEIVED LAST YEAR, I ACHIEVED THIS GOAL IN 12 MONTHS

IT'S OK ALLY
CLIPART & RESOURCES FOR CHILDREN WITH SPECIAL NEEDS

Achievement:
Date this occurred:
How long it took me to reach my goal:
What resources helped me reach my goal?
This new skill has helped me:

THIS IS A PHOTO OF ME ON THE DAY I ACHIEVED MY GOAL

Use the Goodnotes "Add Image" button to add a photo of your achievement below

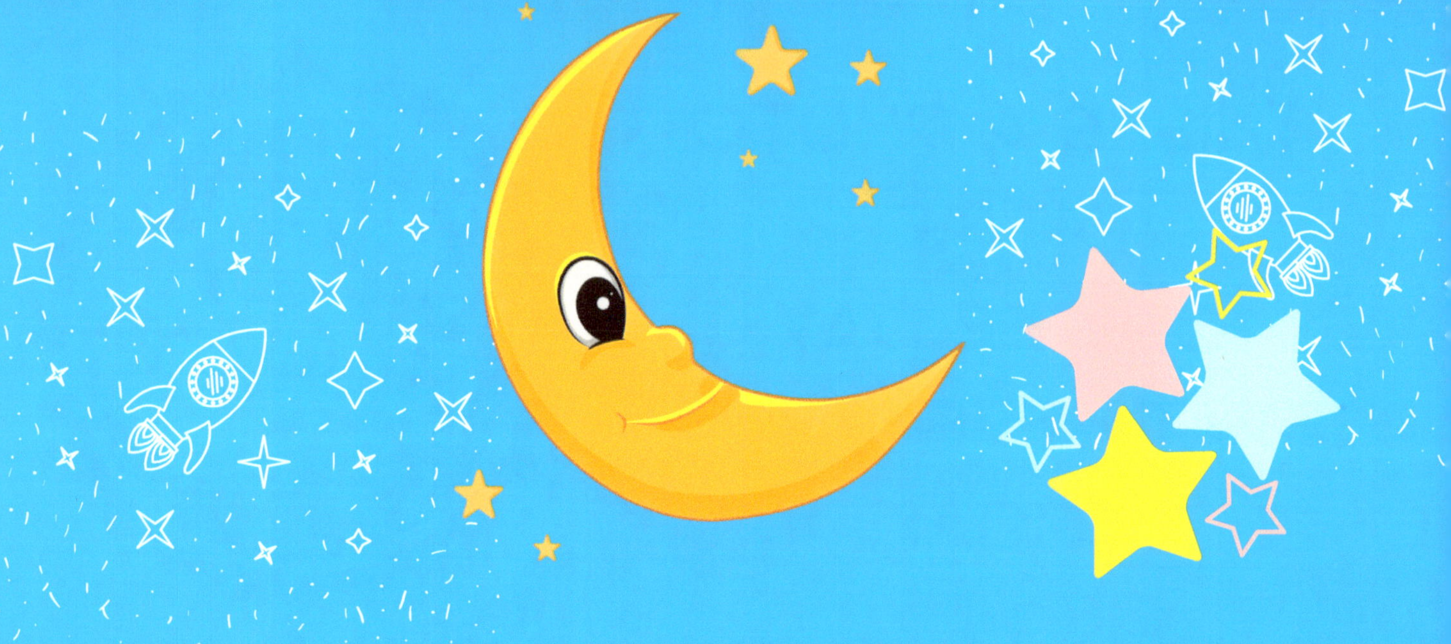

PEOPLE WHO HELP ME REACH MY GOALS

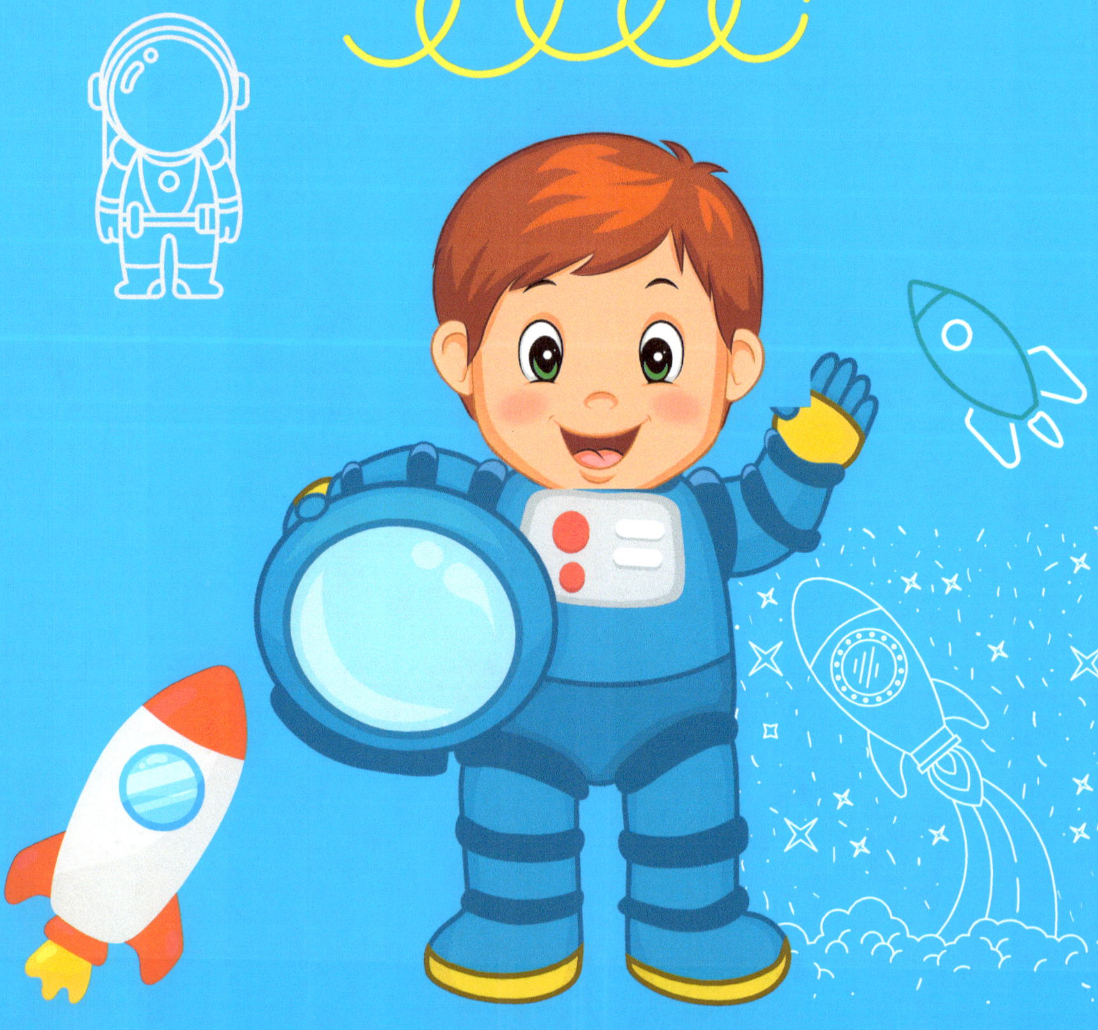

ART THERAPIST PROFESSIONAL

NAME:

PHONE:

EMAIL:

NOTES:

DATE OF REPORT:

KEY POINTS:

	#1	
	#2	
	#3	
	#4	
	#5	
	#6	

ART THERAPIST PROFESSIONAL

Upload screenshots of each page of your report using the photo button in goodnotes and insert into the space below

ART THERAPIST PROFESSIONAL

Upload screenshots of each page of your report using the photo button in goodnotes and insert into the space below

CHIROPRACTOR PROFESSIONAL

NAME:

PHONE:

EMAIL:

NOTES:

DATE OF REPORT:		KEY POINTS:
	#1	
	#2	
	#3	
	#4	
	#5	
	#6	

CHIROPRACTOR PROFESSIONAL

Upload screenshots of each page of your report using the photo button in goodnotes and insert into the space below

CHIROPRACTOR PROFESSIONAL

Upload screenshots of each page of your report using the photo button in goodnotes and insert into the space below

CHIROPRACTOR PROFESSIONAL

Upload screenshots of each page of your report using the photo button in goodnotes and insert into the space below

DiETiCiAN PROFESSIONAL

NAME:

PHONE:

EMAIL:

NOTES:

DATE OF REPORT:		KEY POINTS:
	#1	
	#2	
	#3	
	#4	
	#5	
	#6	

DIETICIAN PROFESSIONAL

Upload screenshots of each page of your report using the photo button in goodnotes and insert into the space below

DIETICIAN PROFESSIONAL

Upload screenshots of each page of your report using the photo button in goodnotes and insert into the space below

DIETICIAN PROFESSIONAL

Upload screenshots of each page of your report using the photo button in goodnotes and insert into the space below

MUSIC THERAPIST PROFESSIONAL

NAME:

PHONE:

EMAIL:

NOTES:

DATE OF REPORT:		KEY POINTS:
	#1	
	#2	
	#3	
	#4	
	#5	
	#6	

MUSIC THERAPIST PROFESSIONAL

Upload screenshots of each page of your report using the photo button in goodnotes and insert into the space below

MUSIC THERAPIST PROFESSIONAL

Upload screenshots of each page of your report using the photo button in goodnotes and insert into the space below

MUSIC THERAPIST PROFESSIONAL

Upload screenshots of each page of your report using the photo button in goodnotes and insert into the space below

NEUROLOGIST REPORT

NAME:

PHONE:

EMAIL:

NOTES:

DATE OF REPORT:		KEY POINTS:
	#1	
	#2	
	#3	
	#4	
	#5	
	#6	

NEUROLOGIST PROFESSIONAL

Upload screenshots of each page of your report using the photo button in goodnotes and insert into the space below

NEUROLOGIST PROFESSIONAL

Upload screenshots of each page of your report using the photo button in goodnotes and insert into the space below

NEUROLOGIST PROFESSIONAL

Upload screenshots of each page of your report using the photo button in goodnotes and insert into the space below

OCCUPATIONAL THERAPIST

NAME:

PHONE:

EMAIL:

NOTES:

DATE OF REPORT:		KEY POINTS:
	#1	
	#2	
	#3	
	#4	
	#5	
	#6	

OCCUPATIONAL THERAPIST REPORT

Upload screenshots of each page of your report using the photo button in goodnotes and insert into the space below

OCCUPATIONAL THERAPIST REPORT

Upload screenshots of each page of your report using the photo button in goodnotes and insert into the space below

OCCUPATIONAL THERAPIST REPORT

Upload screenshots of each page of your report using the photo button in goodnotes and insert into the space below

OPTOMETRIST PROFESSIONAL

NAME:

PHONE:

EMAIL:

NOTES:

DATE OF REPORT:

KEY POINTS:

	#1	
	#2	
	#3	
	#4	
	#5	
	#6	

OPTOMETRIST PROFESSIONAL REPORT

Upload screenshots of each page of your report using the photo button in goodnotes and insert into the space below

OPTOMETRIST PROFESSIONAL REPORT

Upload screenshots of each page of your report using the photo button in goodnotes and insert into the space below

OPTOMETRIST PROFESSIONAL REPORT

Upload screenshots of each page of your report using the photo button in goodnotes and insert into the space below

ORTHOTISTS AND PROSTHETISTS

NAME:

PHONE:

EMAIL:

NOTES:

DATE OF REPORT:		KEY POINTS:
	#1	
	#2	
	#3	
	#4	
	#5	
	#6	

ORTHOTISTS AND PROSTHETISTS PROFESSIONAL

Upload screenshots of each page of your report using the photo button in goodnotes and insert into the space below

ORTHOTISTS AND PROSTHETISTS PROFESSIONAL

Upload screenshots of each page of your report using the photo button in goodnotes and insert into the space below

ORTHOTISTS AND PROSTHETISTS PROFESSIONAL

Upload screenshots of each page of your report using the photo button in goodnotes and insert into the space below

OSTEOTHERAPIST PROFESSIONAL

NAME:

PHONE:

EMAIL:

NOTES:

DATE OF REPORT:

KEY POINTS:

	#1	
	#2	
	#3	
	#4	
	#5	
	#6	

OSTEOTHERAPIST PROFESSIONAL REPORT

Upload screenshots of each page of your report using the photo button in goodnotes and insert into the space below

OSTEOTHERAPIST PROFESSIONAL REPORT

Upload screenshots of each page of your report using the photo button in goodnotes and insert into the space below

OSTEOTHERAPIST PROFESSIONAL REPORT

Upload screenshots of each page of your report using the photo button in goodnotes and insert into the space below

PAEDIATRICIAN REPORT

NAME:

PHONE:

EMAIL:

NOTES:

DATE OF REPORT:

KEY POINTS:

	#1	
	#2	
	#3	
	#4	
	#5	
	#6	

PAEDETRICIAN REPORT

Upload screenshots of each page of your report using the photo button in goodnotes and insert into the space below

PAEDETRICIAN REPORT

Upload screenshots of each page of your report using the photo button in goodnotes and insert into the space below

PAEDETRICIAN REPORT

Upload screenshots of each page of your report using the photo button in goodnotes and insert into the space below

PHYSIOTHERAPIST PROFESSIONAL

NAME:

PHONE:

EMAIL:

NOTES:

DATE OF REPORT:		KEY POINTS:
	#1	
	#2	
	#3	
	#4	
	#5	
	#6	

PHYSIOTHERAPIST PROFESSIONAL REPORT

Upload screenshots of each page of your report using the photo button in goodnotes and insert into the space below

PHYSIOTHERAPIST PROFESSIONAL REPORT

Upload screenshots of each page of your report using the photo button in goodnotes and insert into the space below

PHYSIOTHERAPIST PROFESSIONAL REPORT

Upload screenshots of each page of your report using the photo button in goodnotes and insert into the space below

PODIATRIST PROFESSIONAL

NAME:

PHONE:

EMAIL:

NOTES:

DATE OF REPORT:		KEY POINTS:
	#1	
	#2	
	#3	
	#4	
	#5	
	#6	

PODIATRIST PROFESSIONAL REPORT

Upload screenshots of each page of your report using the photo button in goodnotes and insert into the space below

PODIATRIST PROFESSIONAL REPORT

Upload screenshots of each page of your report using the photo button in goodnotes and insert into the space below

PODIATRIST PROFESSIONAL REPORT

Upload screenshots of each page of your report using the photo button in goodnotes and insert into the space below

PSYCHIATRIST PROFESSIONAL

NAME:

PHONE:

EMAIL:

NOTES:

DATE OF REPORT:		KEY POINTS:
	#1	
	#2	
	#3	
	#4	
	#5	
	#6	

PSYCHIATRIST PROFESSIONAL REPORT

Upload screenshots of each page of your report using the photo button in goodnotes and insert into the space below

PSYCHIATRIST PROFESSIONAL REPORT

Upload screenshots of each page of your report using the photo button in goodnotes and insert into the space below

PSYCHIATRIST PROFESSIONAL REPORT

Upload screenshots of each page of your report using the photo button in goodnotes and insert into the space below

PSYCHOLOGIST PROFESSIONAL

NAME:

PHONE:

EMAIL:

NOTES:

DATE OF REPORT:		KEY POINTS:
	#1	
	#2	
	#3	
	#4	
	#5	
	#6	

PSYCHOLOGIST PROFESSIONAL REPORT

Upload screenshots of each page of your report using the photo button in goodnotes and insert into the space below

PSYCHOLOGIST PROFESSIONAL REPORT

Upload screenshots of each page of your report using the photo button in goodnotes and insert into the space below

PSYCHOLOGIST PROFESSIONAL REPORT

Upload screenshots of each page of your report using the photo button in goodnotes and insert into the space below

SPEECH PATHOLOGIST

NAME:

PHONE:

EMAIL:

NOTES:

DATE OF REPORT:		KEY POINTS:
	#1	
	#2	
	#3	
	#4	
	#5	
	#6	

SPEECH PATHOLOGIST REPORT

Upload screenshots of each page of your report using the photo button in goodnotes and insert into the space below

SPEECH PATHOLOGIST REPORT

Upload screenshots of each page of your report using the photo button in goodnotes and insert into the space below

SPEECH PATHOLOGIST REPORT

Upload screenshots of each page of your report using the photo button in goodnotes and insert into the space below

SOCIAL WORKER PROFESSIONAL

NAME:

PHONE:

EMAIL:

NOTES:

DATE OF REPORT:		KEY POINTS:
	#1	
	#2	
	#3	
	#4	
	#5	
	#6	

SOCIAL WORKER PROFESSIONAL

Upload screenshots of each page of your report using the photo button in goodnotes and insert into the space below

SOCIAL WORKER PROFESSIONAL

Upload screenshots of each page of your report using the photo button in goodnotes and insert into the space below

SOCIAL WORKER PROFESSIONAL

Upload screenshots of each page of your report using the photo button in goodnotes and insert into the space below

SUPPORT WORKER PROFESSIONAL

NAME:

PHONE:

EMAIL:

NOTES:

DATE OF REPORT:		KEY POINTS:
	#1	
	#2	
	#3	
	#4	
	#5	
	#6	

SUPPORT WORKER PROFESSIONAL

Upload screenshots of each page of your report using the photo button in goodnotes and insert into the space below

SUPPORT WORKER PROFESSIONAL

Upload screenshots of each page of your report using the photo button in goodnotes and insert into the space below

SUPPORT WORKER PROFESSIONAL

Upload screenshots of each page of your report using the photo button in goodnotes and insert into the space below

www.ingramcontent.com/pod-product-compliance
Lightning Source LLC
LaVergne TN
LVHW070948210926
848482LV00002B/137
9780645064155